DIGITAL IMAGING IN DIAGNOSTIC RADIOLOGY

DIGITAL IMAGING IN DIAGNOSTIC RADIOLOGY

Edited by

John D. Newell, Jr., M.D., F.C.C.P.

Thoracic Radiologist
Radiological Imaging Associates
Englewood, Colorado
Former Associate Professor and
Chief, Section of Thoracic Radiology
Department of Radiology
University of New Mexico School of Medicine
Albuquerque, New Mexico

and

Charles A. Kelsey, Ph.D., F.A.C.R.

Professor
Department of Radiology
University of New Mexico School of Medicine
Albuquerque, New Mexico

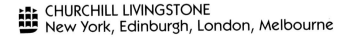

CHURCHILL LIVINGSTONE
New York, Edinburgh, London, Melbourne

Library of Congress Cataloging-in-Publication Data

Digital imaging in diagnostic radiology / edited by John D. Newell,
  Jr., and Charles A. Kelsey.
     p. cm.
   Includes bibliographical references.
   Includes index.
   ISBN 0-443-08634-6
   1. Diagnostic imaging—Digital techniques.   I. Newell, John D.
  II. Kelsey, Charles A.
   [DNLM: 1. Diagnostic Imaging—methods. 2. Technology, Radiologic-
  -methods. WN 200 D5743]
   RC78-7.D53D537 1990
   616.07'57—dc20
   DNLM/DLC
   for Library of Congress   90-2231
                                               CIP

© **Churchill Livingstone Inc. 1990**

Distributed in the United Kingdom by Churchill Livingstone, Robert Stevenson House, 1–3
Baxter's Place, Leith Walk, Edinburgh EH1 3AF, and by associated companies, branches, and
representatives throughout the world.

Accurate indications, adverse reactions, and dosage schedules for drugs are provided in this book,
but it is possible that they may change. The reader is urged to review the package information data
of the manufacturers of the medications mentioned.

The Publishers have made every effort to trace the copyright holders for borrowed material. If
they have inadvertently overlooked any, they will be pleased to make the necessary arrangements
at the first opportunity.

Acquisitions Editor: *Robert A. Hurley*
Copy Editor: *Kathleen P. Lyons*
Production Designer: *Gloria Brown*
Production Supervisor: *Sharon Tuder*

Printed in the United States of America

First published in 1990

Contributors

Stephen Balter, Ph.D.

Senior Medical Physicist, Philips Medical Systems North America, Shelton, Connecticut; Adjunct Associate Professor of Physics, Department of Radiology, Cornell University Medical College, New York, New York

Laurie L. Fajardo, M.D.

Assistant Professor, and Director, Division of Mammography and Breast Imaging, Department of Radiology, University of Arizona College of Medicine, Arizona Health Sciences Center, Tucson, Arizona

Tim B. Hunter, M.D.

Professor, and Director, Division of Body Imaging, Department of Radiology, University of Arizona College of Medicine, Arizona Health Sciences Center; Director, Tucson Breast Center, Tucson, Arizona

Charles A. Kelsey, Ph.D., F.A.C.R.

Professor, Department of Radiology, University of New Mexico School of Medicine, Albuquerque, New Mexico

Jerry N. King, M.D.

Assistant Professor, Department of Radiology, University of New Mexico School of Medicine; Chief, Division of Vascular and Interventional Radiology, Department of Radiology, University of New Mexico Hospital, Albuquerque, New Mexico

Anthony R. Lubinsky, Ph.D.

Research Associate, Eastman Kodak Company, Rochester, New York

John D. Newell, Jr., M.D., F.C.C.P.

Thoracic Radiologist, Radiological Imaging Associates, Englewood, Colorado; Former Associate Professor, and Chief, Section of Thoracic Radiology, Department of Radiology, University of New Mexico School of Medicine, Albuquerque, New Mexico

James F. Owen, Ph.D.

Laboratory Head, Eastman Kodak Company, Rochester, New York

Ralph Schaetzing, Ph.D.

Research Associate, Eastman Kodak Company, Rochester, New York

Wayne T. Stockburger, M.B.A., R.T.R.

Administrative Director, Diagnostic Imaging Services, Alton Ochsner Medical Foundation, New Orleans, Louisiana

Bruce R. Whiting, Ph.D.

Research Associate, Eastman Kodak Company, Rochester, New York

Preface

Digital Imaging in Diagnostic Radiology is intended to provide a basic clinical and technical perspective on digital radiology for anyone interested in the subject. This includes practicing radiologists, radiology residents, engineers and scientists in the field of digital imaging, radiologic technologists, and radiology business managers. The subject of digital radiology covers a large amount of clinical and technical information. The purpose of this work is to give interested parties an insight into current state of the art digital radiology. The book is not intended as a comprehensive review of the entire subject. A shorter monograph dealing with the current successes and limitations of digital imaging in radiology is thought to be more appropriate by the authors because of the limited number of digital radiology systems in clinical operation in the United States today.

The first four chapters discuss the current state of clinical digital radiology. To date the most successful area in digital imaging is digital cinefluoroscopy and angiography. The use of high temporal and spatial resolution systems with road mapping capability is crucial in the practice of neuroradiology, peripheral vascular angiography, and interventional angiography. Potential applications of digital radiology techniques in thoracic, genitourinary, gastrointestinal, and breast radiology are discussed next. While it appears that there is no clear cut indication for a digital system in these organ systems at this time, these chapters emphasize the current level of performance of available prototype digital systems. It is important to recognize that there has been a major advance in conventional radiology imaging with the development of the advanced multiple beam equalization radiography (AMBER) technology. New developments in conventional imaging must be incorporated into any new digital system. Some of the advantages of the digital imaging systems are achieved in the newer AMBER method. The one area of widespread practical application of digital radiology techniques in radiology is teleradiology. This is an area where the advantages of digital teleradiology have encouraged the use of digital techniques in many private radiology practices.

The next portion of the book deals with the technical aspects of digital radiology. The technical issues that must be considered in replacing conventional screen-film radiology with digital radiology techniques are discussed in some detail. It is interesting to note that there are many physical similarities between the phosphors in use in conventional radiology screens and the phosphors that are thought to be the most likely to replace the conventional system in the future. These chapters should familiarize the reader with the important technologies to watch in the future as practical digital radiology systems develop. Data compression is discussed as a separate issue. It is exciting to think that, as major breakthroughs are achieved in the effectiveness of data compression, affordable digital radiology systems will become more available for everyday clinical practice.

The final chapter of the book discusses the economics of converting from a conventional radiology department to an all-digital department. This is one of the major problems in developing digital radiology departments. In this chapter the economic viability of converting to an all-digital radiology format is shown to be more realistic for the large radiology department. Presently, it is not economically feasible for a medium or small radiology department to anticipate conversion to an all-digital format whereas the larger departments may be able to achieve this conversion with a favorable economic result.

John D. Newell, Jr., M.D., F.C.C.P.
Charles A. Kelsey, Ph.D., F.A.C.R.

Contents

CLINICAL
APPLICATIONS

1

Portable Digital Subtraction Angiography

Jerry N. King

INTRODUCTION

The advantages of digital subtraction angiography (DSA) over conventional screen-film angiography include shorter examination time, lower contrast volume, lower cost per examination, higher contrast resolution, and increased patient comfort and safety.[1,2] The accuracy of DSA for evaluating various arterial systems has been documented.[1-3] Portable equipment is now available that allows performance of high quality DSA in a wide range of clinical situations and hospital locations outside the radiology department, including the operating room, the emergency department, and the intensive care unit.[4,5] This chapter describes the portable DSA equipment, its technical features, and its clinical applications, including techniques used in performing portable DSA, accuracy and repetition rate, practical limitations, and cost. Examples of various types of procedures performed with the portable equipment are also shown.

PORTABLE DSA EQUIPMENT: TECHNICAL FEATURES

A mobile DSA C-arm system (OEC-Diasonics, Salt Lake City) with a rotating anode is now commercially available. The system consists of a microprocessor-controlled x-ray mainframe with integrated real-time digital image processing, and a dual-screen monitor. The x-ray tube has a 0.3-mm focal spot, which is small enough to allow acquisition of good quality angiographic images. The rotating anode design increases the heat capacity of the x-ray tube significantly. A kilovolt peak (kVp) of 40 to 120 and a milliampere (mA) current of 2.5 to 5.0 with a 20-mA boost capability may be selected. Fluoroscopy is performed at lower milliamperage, and the milliampere boost is used during angiography. The imaging system includes a high resolution television camera with 360-degree motorized rotation, rotating collimators, either a 6- or a 9-inch input screen, and an image storage system with both a videocassette recorder and a videodisc recorder. The input screen has a central spatial resolution of a 4.4 line pairs per millimeter (lp/mm) and a peripheral spatial resolution of a 3.6 lp/mm with a 512 × 512 image matrix. The unit can be powered from any 115-volt, 20-ampere electrical outlet. The system allows real-time subtraction at 30 frames per second. This fast frame rate eliminates flicker so that contrast is visualized flowing smoothly through vessels. Images can be viewed either subtracted or nonsubtracted. Other features of the system include digital window and level controls, frame averaging, road mapping, and peak opacification. Road mapping and peak opacification are particularly helpful during complex angiographic procedures in which subselective catheterization must be performed.

PORTABLE DSA: TECHNIQUES

Performance of angiography outside the radiology department obviously requires the availability not only of portable DSA x-ray equipment but also of ancillary equipment. Therefore, a separate cart capable of carrying catheters, guide wires, stopcocks, sterile gloves, sterile gowns and drapes, and all the other equipment necessary for performing angiography must be readily available and consistently restocked. An appropriate-sized supply cart, the mobile C-arm and monitor cart, and a portable power injector are transported to the angiography site. All these components will fit into a standard-size elevator in one load.

Examinations in the operating room are performed on a radiolucent operating table. For neurosurgical patients an initial localizing angiogram is obtained with the patient under general anesthesia. Femoral artery access is maintained during neurosurgery with a vascular sheath, which is infused with heparinized saline flush solution on microdrip. Angiogra-

phy can then be repeated as often as necessary in the operating room until a satisfactory surgical end point is reached. This technique is especially useful during surgery for intracranial aneurysms and vascular malformations. Figures 1-1 to 1-3 are examples of intraoperative angiograms performed with the mobile DSA system.

Immediate surgery to stop life-threatening hemorrhage is necessary in some trauma patients. With the portable C-arm unit, these patients can undergo angiography in the operating room instead of being awakened from general anesthesia and transported to the radiology department. In patients who have critical intra-abdominal hemorrhage but also have suspected vascular injuries in the extremities, this technique is especially useful.

Examinations in the emergency department and intensive care unit can be performed on a radiolucent nuclear medicine imaging table or on a stretcher that has been designed for use with a C-arm. The C-arm stretcher has a sliding radiolucent table top, which can be raised or lowered. Protective aprons must be worn by persons performing the angiography and by persons caring for the patient. In general, no other special shielding is necessary. This has been documented by radiation dose measurements performed with phantoms and by radiation dose monitoring of emergency department personnel.[6] Table 1-1 summarizes typical radiation levels in coulombs per kilogram per hour and milliroentgens per hour during an emergency department DSA examination. These values were obtained at angiographic exposure levels, that is, entrance expo-

Table 1-1 Typical Radiation Levels From An Emergency Department DSA Examination

Distance from Patient (cm)	Scattered Radiation Level	
	$C\ kg^{-1}\ hr^{-1}$	$mR\ hr^{-1}$
50	5.2×10^{-5}	200
100	2.6×10^{-5}	100
200	7.7×10^{-6}	30
1,000	5.2×10^{-7}	2

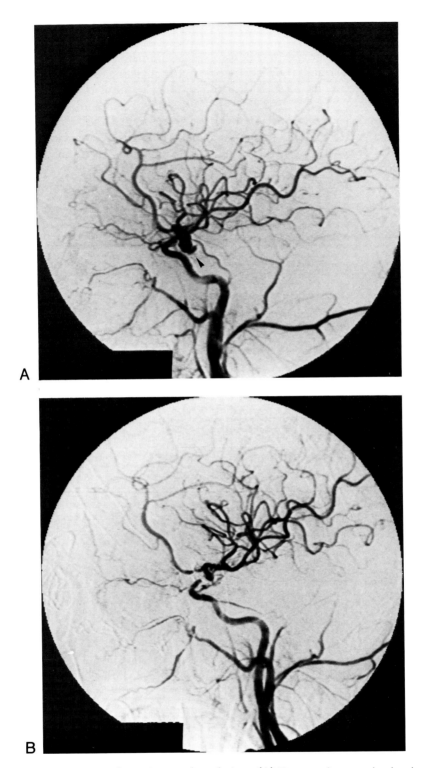

Fig. 1-1. Intraoperative carotid arteriogram, lateral view. **(A)** Preoperative examination in operating room demonstrates posterior communicating artery aneurysm (arrow). **(B)** Intraoperative DSA reveals successful clipping of aneurysm and patency of adjacent vessels.

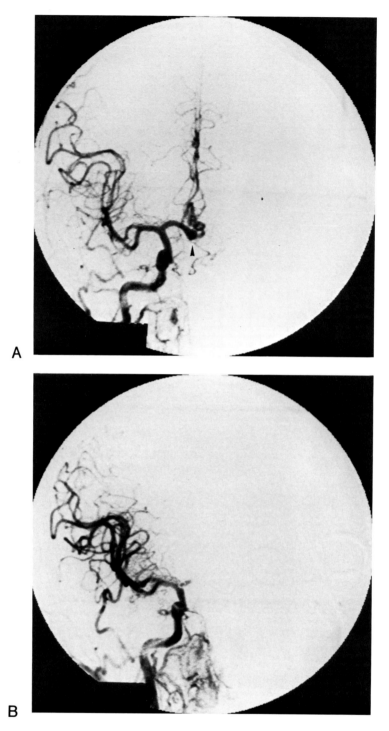

Fig. 1-2. (A) Right carotid injection (posteroanterior projection) performed in operating room reveals aneurysm of anterior communicating artery (arrow). **(B)** Intraoperative DSA performed immediately after aneurysm clipping reveals absence of flow in anterior cerebral arteries. *(Figure continues.)*

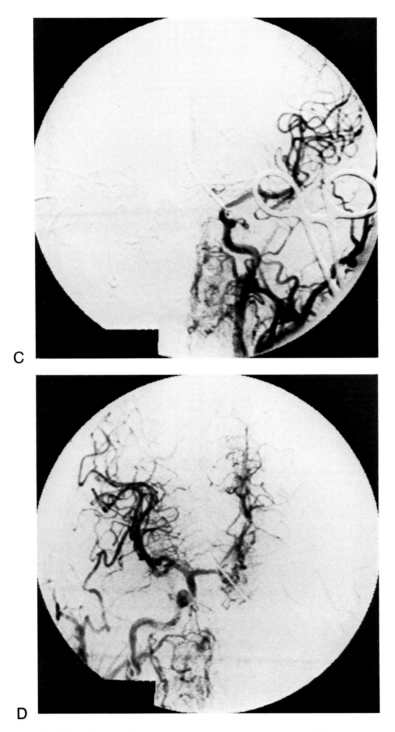

Fig. 1-2 *(Continued)*. **(C)** Left carotid injection (posteroanterior projection) also reveals no flow in anterior cerebral arteries. **(D)** Intraoperative DSA performed after removal of aneurysm clip reveals restoration of flow in anterior cerebral arteries.

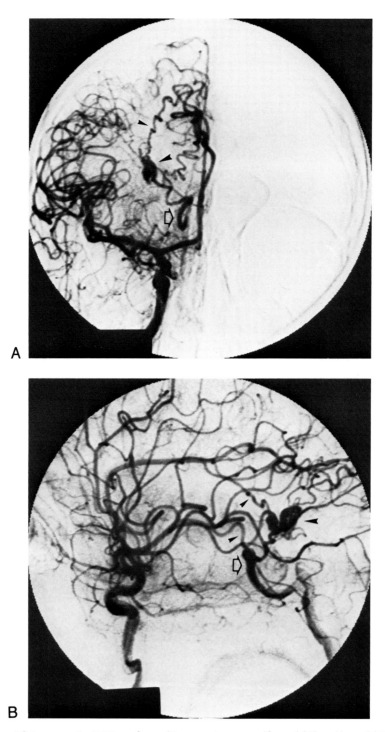

Fig. 1-3. (A & B) Preoperative DSA performed in operating room (frontal **(A)** and lateral **(B)** projections) demonstrates arteriovenous malformation (large arrows) deep in parietal lobe. Note large feeding arteries (small arrows) and early draining vein (open arrows). *(Figure continues.)*

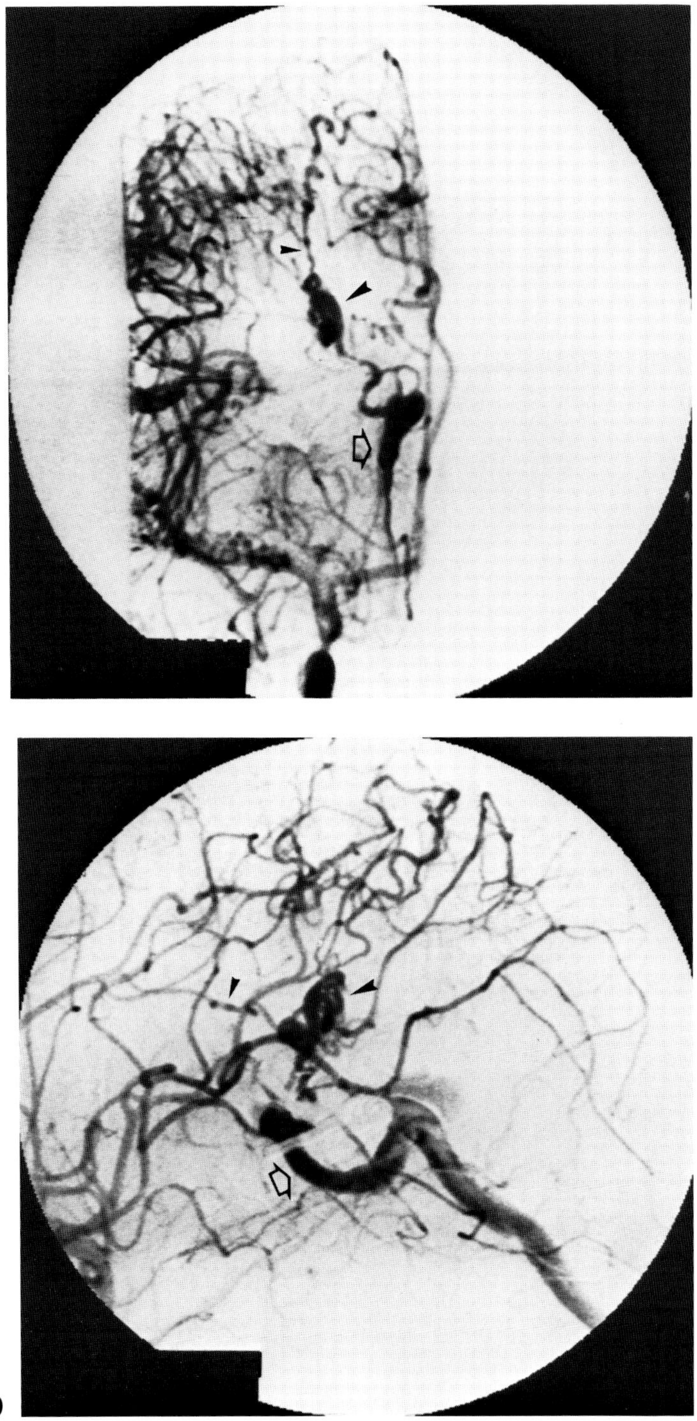

Fig. 1-3 *(Continued).* **(C & D)** Intraoperative DSA (frontal **(C)** and lateral **(D)** projections) performed after several hours of surgery reveals persistent arteriovenous malformation nidus (large arrows) with large feeding arteries (small arrows) and early draining vein (open arrows). *(Figure continues.)*

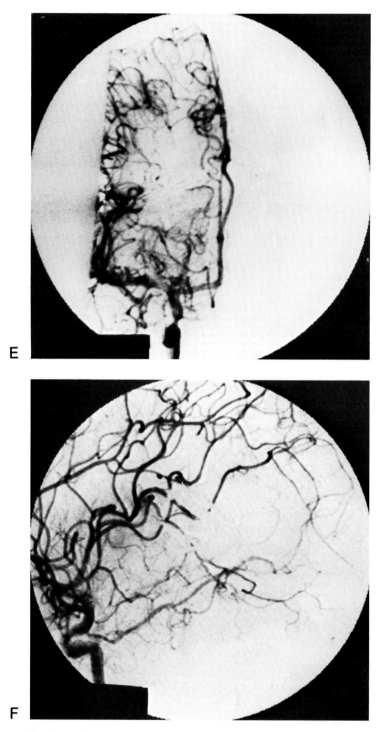

Fig. 1-3 *(Continued).* **(E & F)** Intraoperative carotid DSA (frontal **(E)** and lateral **(F)** projections) performed following further surgery reveals successful resection of AVM.

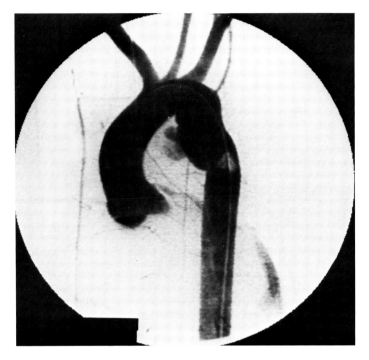

Fig. 1-4. Thoracic aortogram performed with portable DSA equipment reveals transected aorta in a trauma patient.

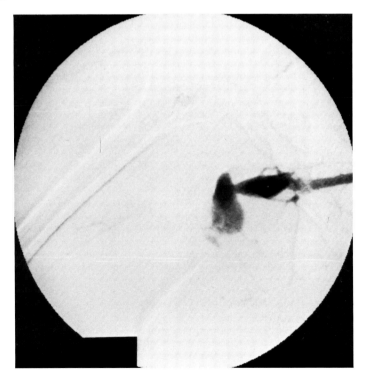

Fig. 1-5. DSA performed in the emergency department on an automobile accident victim reveals avulsion of right axillary artery with extravasation of contrast into soft tissues of axilla.

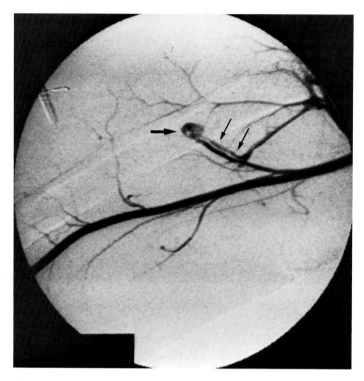

Fig. 1-6. DSA performed with portable equipment reveals false aneurysm (large arrow) and arteriovenous fistula in a patient who was stabbed in the arm. Note abnormal venous opacification during arterial phase (small arrows).

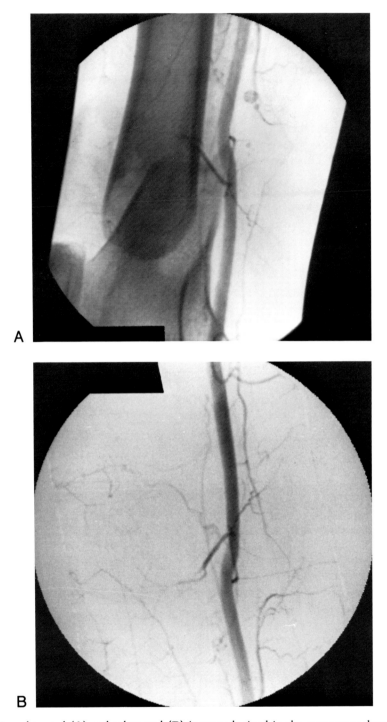

Fig. 1-7. Nonsubtracted **(A)** and subtracted **(B)** images obtained in the emergency department reveal fractured distal femur, with displacement of adjacent artery but no evidence of arterial injury.

sure rates of 1.4×10^{-2} C kg^{-1}min^{-1} (56 R min^{-1}). Entrance exposure levels during fluoroscopy were 2.3×10^{-3} C kg^{-1}min^{-1} (8.8 R min^{-1}).

Use of portable DSA equipment for angiography in the emergency department can significantly decrease the average time interval from patient arrival in the emergency department to completion of arteriograms.[4] This is due in part to the fact that many diagnostic and therapeutic procedures that are usually performed prior to transferring the patient to the radiology department can be performed while the equipment is being readied and while the angiogram is in progress; it is also due in part to the elimination of multiple patient transfers. One can only assume that the time saved is beneficial to the patient. The use of portable DSA equipment in the intensive care unit allows angiographic examination of critically ill and unstable patients, of whom many are encumbered by a host of monitoring equipment and personnel and require moment to moment changes in therapy and life support systems, without moving them from the intensive care unit environment or interrupting their critical care.

PORTABLE DSA: ACCURACY, LIMITATIONS, COST

Portable DSA equipment has been used for angiography in most commonly examined areas of the body with a high degree of accuracy. In one series begun in June 1987 at the University of New Mexico Hospital, 300 consecutive diagnostic angiograms were obtained with portable DSA equipment, and a repeat examination by conventional technique was necessary in only two of these cases (0.7 percent). Figures 1-4 through 1-11 illustrate arteriograms obtained with portable DSA equipment. The equipment can also be used for embolotherapy and thrombolytic therapy patients, as well as for those requiring general radiologic intervention (see Fig. 1-12).

There are only two significant disadvantages or limitations to the use of portable as compared with fixed DSA equipment. The first disadvantage is the relatively small field size. For some types of examinations one or two more contrast injections may be necessary than would be required with a larger image intensifier, which may lengthen the procedure slightly. While the small additional volume of contrast could theoretically be detrimental to patients with borderline or abnormal renal function, the incidence of complications so far has been no greater with portable DSA equipment than with fixed equipment.[4]

The other limitation is one that is common to all DSA equipment. Motion, either of the entire patient or of organs in the imaging field, can result in registration artifacts, which can significantly degrade the quality of digital subtraction images. This is most important in the chest, where cardiac and respiratory motion can degrade image quality, and in the abdomen, where image quality can be degraded by peristalsis or respiratory movement of gas-filled bowel. Therefore conventional film-screen angiography is the technique of choice for pulmonary arteriography and is sometimes required for good quality gastrointestinal and renal angiography.

The cost of portable DSA equipment depends on the type of equipment purchased. Depending on the type of fixed equipment used for comparison, the cost of portable DSA equipment is estimated to be between 10 and 20 percent of the cost of purchasing and installing an angiographic room with fixed DSA equipment.

SUMMARY

Portable DSA equipment can be used to provide rapid, accurate angiographic information in a wide range of clinical situations and hospital locations. Although the technique has some limitations, it is a useful adjunct in the evaluation of vascular disease and in some cases may be a cost-effective alternative to conventional angiography with fixed equipment.

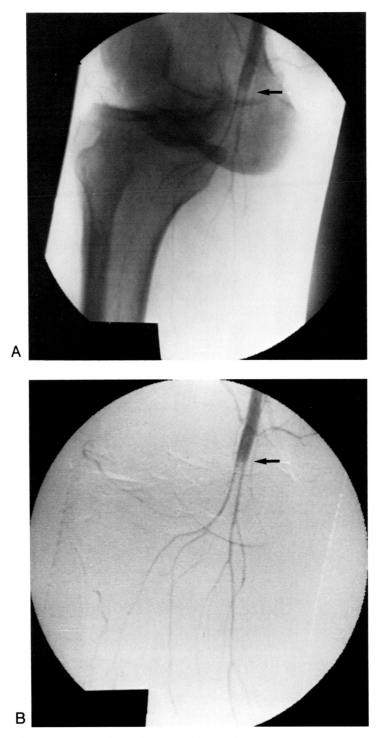

Fig. 1-8. Same leg as in Fig. 1-7. Nonsubtracted **(A)** and subtracted **(B)** images reveal total occlusion of the popliteal artery at the level of the knee joint (arrow).

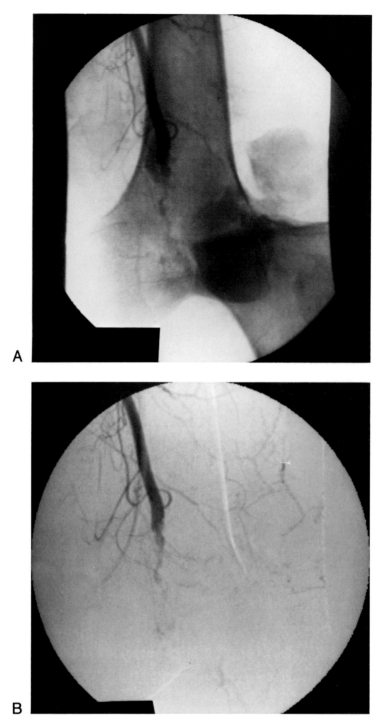

Fig. 1-9. Same patient as in Figs. 1-7 and 1-8, opposite leg. Nonsubtracted **(A)** and subtracted **(B)** images reveal knee dislocation and total occlusion of the popliteal artery. All of this patient's arteriograms were obtained in the emergency department with portable DSA equipment.

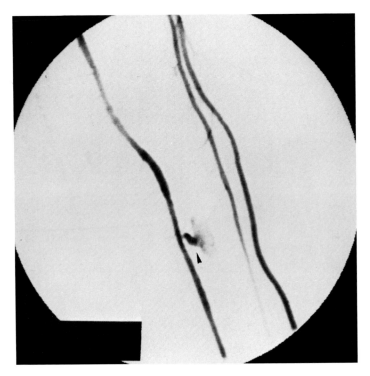

Fig. 1-10. Patient with fractured tibia. DSA performed with portable equipment reveals extravasation of contrast from injured posterior tibial artery (arrow).

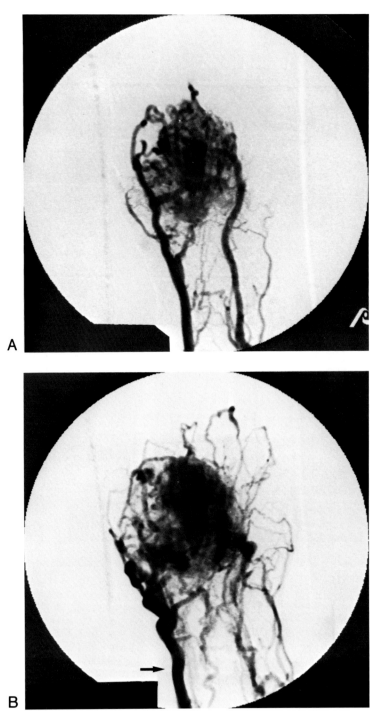

Fig. 1-11. Arteriovenous malformation of hand. **(A)** Early arterial phase reveals markedly enlarged radial and ulnar arteries supplying abnormal tangle of vessels in palm. **(B)** Midarterial phase reveals further opacification of the arteriovenous malformation with large early draining vein (arrow). Note the absence of detectable flow into digital arteries.

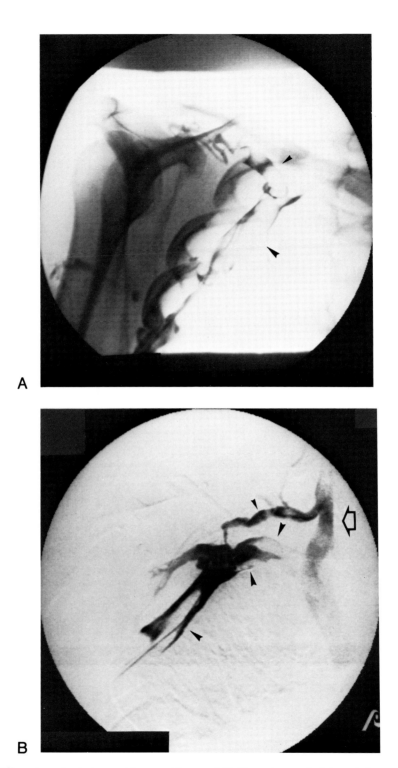

Fig. 1-12. Effort thrombosis in an 18-year-old man. **(A)** Nonsubtracted right subclavian venogram reveals thrombus in subclavian vein (large arrowhead) and in large collateral vein (small arrowhead). **(B)** Digital subtraction venogram after 18 hours of thrombolytic therapy with urokinase infusion directly into clot reveals residual thrombus (large arrowheads). Note collateral vein (small arrowhead) draining into the internal jugular vein (open arrow). *(Figure continues.)*

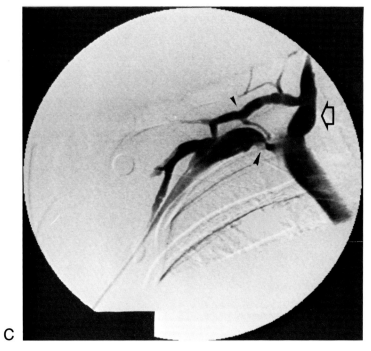

C

Fig. 1-12 *(Continued).* **(C)** Digital subtraction venogram following 23 hours of thrombolytic therapy. Thrombus has been completely dissolved. Note severe stenosis of subclavian vein (large arrow) and collateral venous drainage (small arrow) into internal jugular vein (open arrow) and superior vena cava.

REFERENCES

1. Mirvis S, Pais S, Gens D: Thoracic aortic rupture: Advantages of intra-arterial digital subtraction angiography. AJR 146:987, 1986
2. Weinstein M, Pavlicek W, Modic M, Duchesneau P: Intra-arterial digital subtraction angiography of the head and neck. Radiology 147:717, 1983
3. Sibbit R, Palmaz J, Garcia F, Reuter S: Trauma of the extremities: Prospective comparison of digital and conventional angiography. Radiology 160:179, 1986
4. King JN, Orrison WM, Keck GM, et al: Arteriography with portable DSA equipment. Radiology 172:1023, 1989
5. Hieshima GB, Reicher MA, Higashida RT, et al: Intraoperative digital subtraction neuroangiography: A diagnostic and therapeutic tool. AJNR 8:759, 1987
6. Kelsey CA, King JN, Orrison WM, Mettler FA: Scatter radiation levels from a portable fluoroscopic/angiographic unit. Health Phys 57:817, 1989

2

Digital Radiology of the Thorax

John D. Newell, Jr.
Charles A. Kelsey

INTRODUCTION

In modern imaging departments a great many examinations are already performed with use of digital techniques. These include ultrasonography, nuclear radiology, computed tomography (CT), magnetic resonance imaging, digital fluoroscopy, and digital subtraction angiography. It is not surprising that most radiologists and radiologic scientists are also interested in developing viable techniques for other applications of digital radiology. Chest radiography accounts for about 40 percent of the conventional radiographs done in a radiology department. This examination demands high spatial resolution as well as high contrast sensitivity across a wide dynamic range of x-ray exposure to the radiologic detector. The current analog system of conventional radiography is reliable and inexpensive. A new system should offer some combination of cost advantage, increased diagnostic capability, and reliability when compared with existing modern conventional radiography systems. In this chapter we review the leading technologies for a replacement digital radiography system.

Filtration devices are necessary on all x-ray tube sources in order to reduce the amount of low energy radiation that the patient is exposed to but that does not contribute to formation of the radiologic image. Additional filtration of the x-ray beam by shaped filters has been used to increase the quality of the final radiologic image of the chest[1-3] by attenuating the x-ray beam more in the area of the lungs and less in the area of the cardiomediastinal structures.

The difficulty that arises in using a shaped filter system is the large variation in the shape and contents of the thorax in different patients. The most sophisticated application of this methodology is the digital beam attenuator developed at the University of Wisconsin.[4,5] A patient-specific filter is formed by first scanning the chest to determine the attenua-

21

tion pattern of the x-ray beam over the thorax. This information is used to generate a metallic cerium impregnated ribbon which is then placed in front of the x-ray tube prior to obtaining the final radiograph. This is still a laboratory concept, and a clinical prototype is not in operation at this time.

The grid-detector combination must record meaningful information regarding the thorax in the areas of the mediastinum, lung, and chest wall. If one uses a 120-kVp grid technique (12:1 grid ratio), the ratio of scatter to primary radiation is 1.3:1 in the lung and 2.3:1 in the mediastinum.[6,10] Less than 50 percent of the subject contrast is utilized in conventional chest radiography even when a grid is used.

The major advantages of existing dedicated chest radiography (DCR) systems are that they are capable of economically providing high quality radiographs of the thorax in most instances and that the film provides a simple and cost-effective way of detecting, displaying, transporting, and storing the radiologic image. The disadvantages of the DCR systems include a limited dynamic range which may preclude diagnosing small nodules or mediastinal disease in some patients. The integration of the detection and display functions into the film make additional retrospective manipulation of the radiologic image with computed image processing impossible, unless the film is digitized.

SCANNING EQUALIZATION RADIOGRAPHY

SER has been developed at several centers including the University of Rochester Medical Center over the past several years.[7-9] In the original University of Rochester SER system,[7] a 3.5 cm collimated beam of x-rays is swept over a 35 × 43 cm film in 4.7 seconds. A collimator is placed between the patient and the screen-film combination to reduce scattered radiation on the image. The x-ray tube is pulsed with a frequency between 1,237 and 1,893 Hz, while the film exposure for each pulse is monitored by a detector behind the film. The detector moves with the aft slit collimator during the scanning process. The duration of every x-ray pulse is adjusted at each beam position to create the optimal film exposure. The resultant image is composed of 6,500 small, overlapping images, which are positioned on the film to avoid scan line artifacts. The adjustment in patient exposure is automatic for each patient to avoid large excursions in film exposure. The basic elements of the SER system are shown in Figure 2-1.

SER and DCR type systems have been compared with one another in two studies.[7,8] In the first study conventional and SER radiographs of normal thoracic anatomy were obtained at 120 kVp with Kodak Lanex medium screens and Kodak Ortho-G film. The conventional system used a 10:1 ratio stationary grid, and the exposures were phototimed. The SER system had a 4.7-second exposure time, 0.33 seconds at any one point. The results of this study indicated that posteroanterior (PA) radiographs obtained with SER provide better visibility of lung detail in the retrocardiac and retrodiaphragmatic regions of the thorax than those obtained with a comparable DCR system. Rib and spine detail were also seen better with the SER system than with conventional radiography.

In this study 12 discrete anatomic features were assessed by six radiologists using both an independent review and a side by side comparison of SER and conventional radiographs. The anatomic features that were assessed were central lung vessels, peripheral lung markings, retrocardiac lung, retrodiaphragmatic lung, trachea, main bronchi, azygoesophageal line, anterior/posterior junction line, aortic contour, ribs, thoracic spine, and heart contour. The SER-produced radiographs were preferred to the conventional radiographs 54 percent of the time, SER was equivalent to standard radiographs 40 percent of the time, and the conventional images were judged superior only 6 percent of the time.[7]

In the second study, SER and conventional

Fig. 2-1. Elements of a scanning equalization radiography (SER) system with slit collimator (**A**) and raster collimator (**B**) configurations. (From Wandtke et al, with permission[7].)

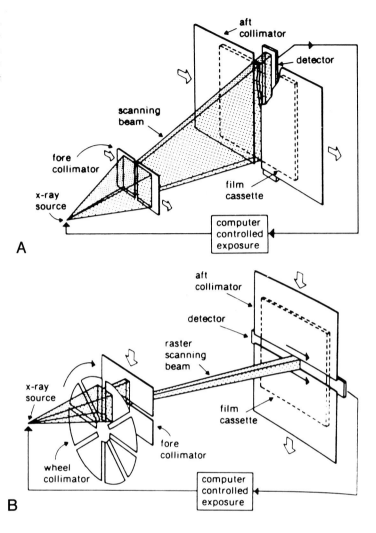

radiography were compared in the evaluation of 95 patients, including 51 normals and 44 abnormals. Both types of radiographs were obtained at 120 kVp with Kodak Lanex medium screens and Kodak Ortho-G film. The conventional system used a 10:1 grid ratio stationary grid, and the exposures were phototimed. The SER system had a 4.7-second exposure time, 0.33 seconds at any one point. The resultant films were all viewed by four radiologists. Abnormalities on the films included alveolar opacities, nodules or mass, interstitial opacities, hilar adenopathy, medias-tinal adenopathy, bony disease, pleural disease, and miscellaneous. The number of true positives increased by 3 percent and the number of true negatives by 9 percent when the SER system was used instead of conventional radiography. This result was statistically significant. Also, 7 percent fewer false positives were seen with SER.[8]

The major criticism of the above two SER studies is that the screen-film combination used was not the optimum one as far as conventional radiography is concerned. A more recent study has been concluded at the University of Rochester[9] comparing the results of eight radiologists using both SER and conventional radiographs. The sensitivity of the SER system was greater, 0.95 compared with 0.92, and the specificity of the SER system was greater, 0.90 compared with 0.75, than for conventional radiography. This study showed that for all diagnostic disease categories the diagnostic accuracy of SER was equal to or greater than that of conventional radiography.

A new development in scanning equalization techniques is a multiple beam scanning equalization radiography (AMBER) system, being developed by the Oldelft Corporation in the Netherlands. This system is similar in principle to the SER system described above, but the AMBER system uses about 20 beams of radiation instead of a single beam.[11] Figure 2-2 illustrates the basic components of the AMBER system. The larger number of beams shortens the scan time and increases the amount of radiation that can be delivered from the system. The use of multiple x-ray beams does not unduly increase the scatter reaching the detector. The multiple beam technology also permits a decrease in x-ray tube loading. The faster scan times and the prolongation of x-ray tube life are two significant advances of the AMBER system over the single beam SER system described above.

Rather than changing the amount of radiation reaching the patient by adjusting the output of the x-ray tube, the AMBER System uses a fan beam which is divided into twenty segments. The intensity of each segment is individually varied to produce an optimal expo-

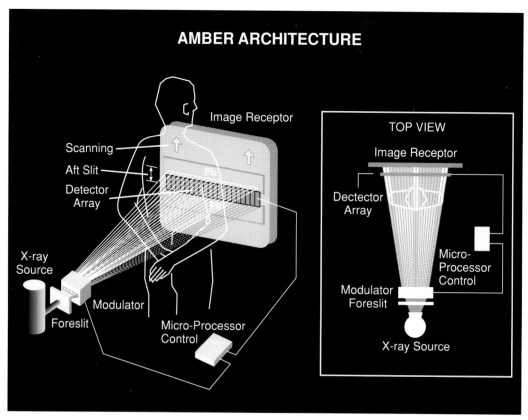

Fig. 2-2. Schematic diagram of the operation of the AMBER exposure equalization system. (Courtesy of Eastman Kodak Company, Rochester, New York.)

Fig. 2-3. (A) Conventional film image of normal male chest. **(B)** AMBER image of normal male chest obtained using a PSP detector demonstrating improved visibility in the retrocardiac and retrosternal areas. *(Figure continues.)*

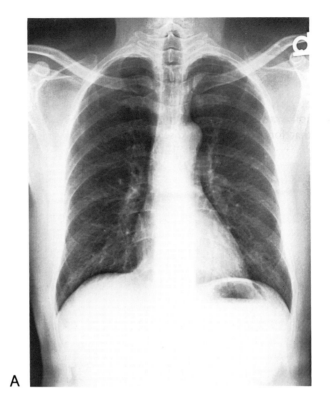

A

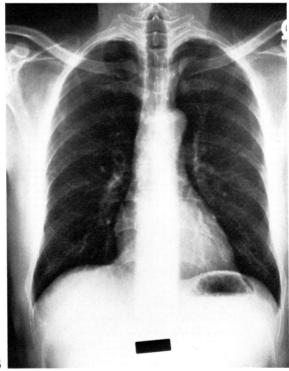

B

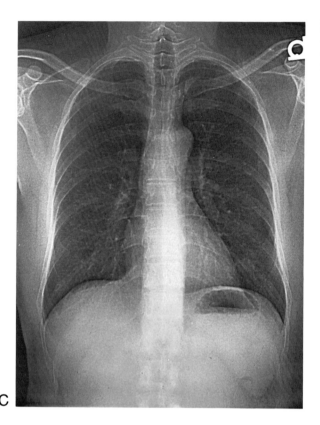

C

Fig. 2-3 *(Continued).* **(C)** AMBER image of normal male chest obtained using a PSP detector processed with edge enhancement. (Courtesy of H.K. Huang, Ph.D.)

sure by positioning a small wedged-shaped attenuator in the modulator. The amount of attenuation is controlled by the detector located behind the patient. The detector array is located in the aft slit between two lead strips designed to prevent scatter radiation from reaching the film or PSP used as the image receptor. The modulator is located close to the x-ray source so the amount of motion of the wedge "fingers" during insertion and removal from the x-ray beam is minimal and the exposure time of the system is adequate. Typical scan times are less than 2 seconds for a 14 × 17 inch chest x-ray. The AMBER system works well when conventional film is used as the image receptor and it works even better with a PSP because the displayed image can be manipulated to enhance or eliminate features.

Early laboratory studies have shown that the AMBER system increases the detection of pulmonary nodules in the lung areas that are superimposed on the mediastinum and dia-

phragm in projection radiography.[11] Figures 2-3 and 2-4 compare normal anatomy images obtained with film to those obtained with AMBER scanning beam system using a PSP image detector system. Figures 2-5, 2-6, and 2-7 illustrate some images obtained with an AMBER imaging system.

DIGITAL IMAGE DETECTORS

A digital image that is acquired by using projection radiography can be described as a two-dimensional array of picture elements, or *pixels.* The size of the object and the number of pixels in the array determine the maximum spatial resolution that can be achieved in the object. The magnitude of the number that can be stored in each individual pixel determines the number of gray levels, or the dynamic range, of x-ray intensities that can be accu-

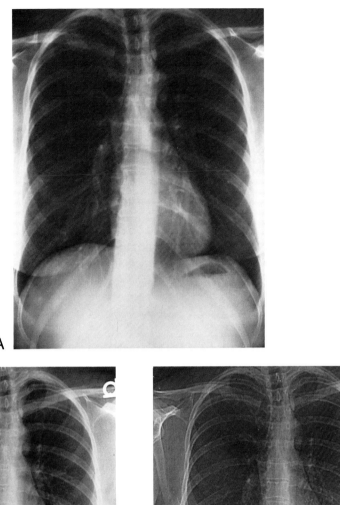

A

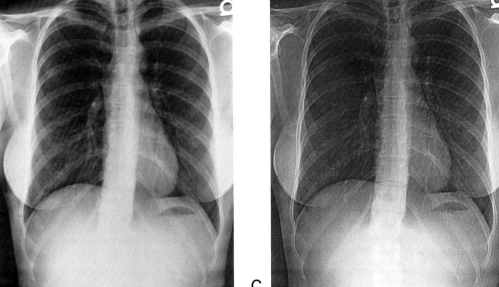

B   C

Fig. 2-4. **(A)** Conventional film image of normal female chest. **(B)** AMBER image of normal female chest obtained using a PSP detector demonstrating the improved visibility in the retrocardiac and retrosternal areas. **(C)** AMBER image of a normal female chest obtained using a PSP detector processed with edge enhancement. (Courtesy of H.K. Huang, Ph.D.)

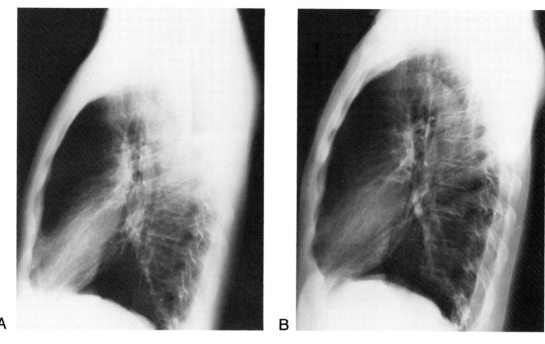

Fig. 2-5. (A) Conventional radiograph of the thorax showing increased retrosternal and retrocardiac film densities. **(B)** Lateral AMBER image demonstrating improved film densities in the retrosternal and retrocardiac areas. (Courtesy of Eastman Kodak Company, Rochester, New York.)

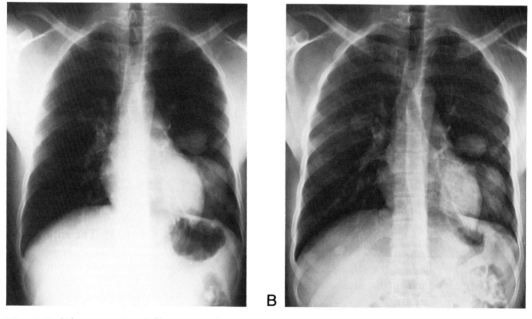

Fig. 2-6. (A) Conventional film image demonstrating the limited visibility of mediastinal and subdiaphragmatic regions. **(B)** AMBER image demonstrating the greater conspicuity of nodules in all areas. (Courtesy of Eastman Kodak Company, Rochester, New York.)

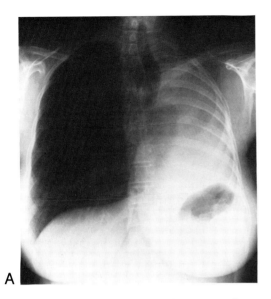

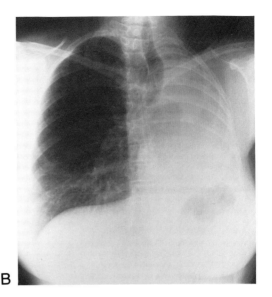

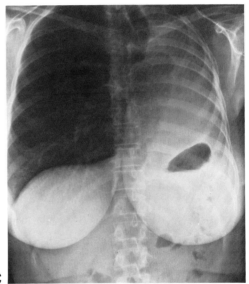

Fig. 2-7. (A) Conventional film image demonstrating collapse of the left lung. Right lung is overpenetrated. **(B)** Conventional film image demonstrating exposure corrected for right lung field. **(C)** AMBER image demonstrating correct equalized image in a single exposure. (Courtesy of Eastman Kodak Company, Rochester, New York.)

rately recorded. Very large ranges of x-ray intensities must be recorded in each pixel so that wide variations in contrast can be preserved in the digital image. However, the pixel array becomes very large if the same spatial resolution is maintained in the digital image as in conventional radiography. It is generally accepted that a pixel array of at least 2048 × 2048 is necessary in a digital image of the chest.[12] The number of discrete x-ray intensi-

ties that are necessary is not quite as clear, but 1024 discrete gray levels can be stored by using only 10 bits ($2^{10} = 1024$). The entire digital image — 2048 × 2048 × 10 bits — will require 8.4 Mbytes of storage. This is quite a lot of information to store, but it is comparable with the storage requirement of a CT study of the thorax. If 20 axial images are obtained to cover the entire thorax as a PA image for a CT array size of 512 × 512 × 11 bits, the CT storage requirement is 11 Mbytes. If frontal and lateral views of the thorax are required, then the amount of information to be stored using CR is 16.8 Mbytes.

These large data storage requirements emphasize the potential importance of data compression in making digital radiography a practical technique in the clinic. The 2048 × 2048 × 10 bit digital image corresponds to a radiograph that has 2.5 line pairs per millimeter (lp/mm) spatial resolution. This modern conventional radiograph will have a minimum of 5.0 lp/mm of spatial resolution. Before a digital system will be accepted by thoracic radiologists, it must preserve the diagnostic ability of the conventional system across a broad number of disease processes and hopefully extend this ability in many diseases of the thorax. The advantages and disadvantages of having a digital image recorded, displayed, transported, and stored in digital format are discussed in subsequent sections.

Digital detector systems have been classified by the geometry of the x-ray beam that they use. These include broad area beam geometry, fan beam geometry, and pencil beam geometry.

Area Beam Geometry

Systems with area beam geometry utilize the same x-ray tubes and collimators as the DCR system described above. These systems include photostimulable phosphors (PSPs), film digitization, and image intensifiers. The advantage of these systems is that they use a large portion of existing equipment from any DCR and have tube heat loads similar to conventional systems. Some of these systems can be easily adapted to do portable radiography.

The PSP system, discussed in detail in Chapter 6, uses an imaging plate (IP) with a PSP coating.[13] The IP is used instead of a conventional screen-film cassette. The latent radiographic image is stored by using the unique properties of the PSP, which is capable of storing energy in a quasi-stable state when excited by x-rays. A PSP-coated IP that has been exposed to x-rays will re-emit luminescent radiation when irradiated with a helium neon laser beam; the luminescent radiation can be recorded by a photomultiplier tube, and the amplified electronic signal is digitized and recorded to produce a digital radiograph with a spatial resolution of 2.5 to 4.0 lp/mm for an adult chest.[6] In children a smaller IP, 20 × 25 cm, can be used, boosting the resolution to 5 lp/mm. The PSP has a linear photoluminescence vs. dose response that is a full order of magnitude greater than that of traditional screen-film systems.

The wide latitude and image processing ability enable the PSP system to record a wide range of exposures. The PSP detector system can be used in portable radiography, and it virtually eliminates any repeat examinations because of its wide dynamic range. Figures 2-8 to 2-10 present examples of PSP portable radiography. It also permits considerable reduction of the dose to pediatric patients with very little loss of image quality. Figures 2-11 to 2-14 are examples of PSP pediatric images.

The PSP system has been shown to be as good as conventional radiography in detecting pulmonary nodules.[13] Figures 2-15 to 2-18 illustrate representative images obtained with such a system. Note that by different processing, information in the lung fields or retrocardiac and retrosternal regions can be displayed. Preliminary results with additional processing of PSP system images suggest that these PSP systems can outperform conventional radiography in the detection of pulmonary nodules. However, a study published in 1989 indicates that some radiologists obtain better results with conventional radiography than with storage phosphor systems in the detection of pneumothorax.[14] This study used a PSP system with a resolution of 2.5 lp/mm and a pixel size of 0.2 × 0.2 mm. Other studies show the storage phosphor system is equal to conventional screen-film systems.[15,16] Further work is needed with the PSP systems at 2.5 lp/mm to determine their performance in other high spatial resolution tasks such as detection of

Fig. 2-8. (A) Female chest image obtained with portable PSP detector and processed to produce a conventional "film" appearance. **(B)** Female chest image obtained with portable PSP detector and processed to improve the visibility of retrosternal and retrocardiac areas. Compare the appearance and visibility of the enlarged heart, congestive heart failure, bilateral pleural effusion and consolidation of the left lower lobe in Figures 2-8 A and B. (Courtesy of S. Balter, Ph.D.)

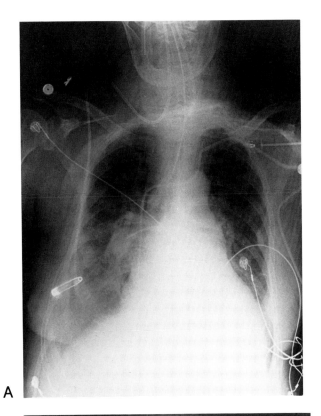

A

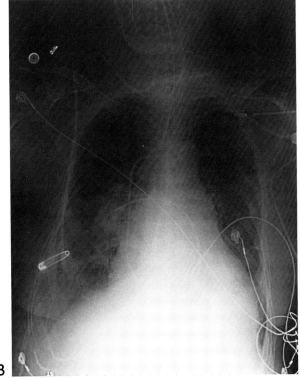

B

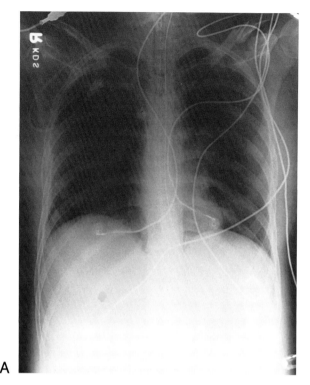

A

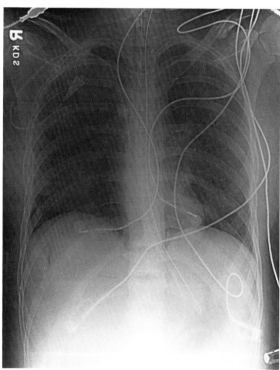

B

Fig. 2-9. **(A)** Chest image obtained with portable PSP detector and processed to produce a conventional film image. **(B)** Same chest image obtained with portable PSP detector processed to improve the visibility of retrosternal and retrocardiac areas. Compare the appearance and visibility of the left upper infiltrate and enlarged left hilum in Figures 2-9A and 2-9B. (Courtesy of S. Balter, Ph.D.)

Fig. 2-10. (A) Chest image obtained with portable PSP detector and processed to produce a "conventional film" image appearance. **(B)** Chest image obtained using a portable PSP detector and processed to improve the visibility of the retrocardiac and retrosternal areas. Note irregular opacities in both lungs that are more confluent in left upper and left lower lung. Compare the appearance and visibility of the left rib fracture, the elevated left hemi-diaphragm, and the infiltrates in Figure 2-10A and B. (Courtesy of S. Balter, Ph.D.)

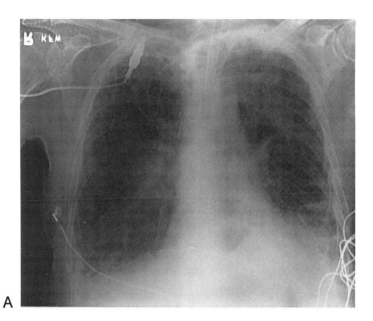

A

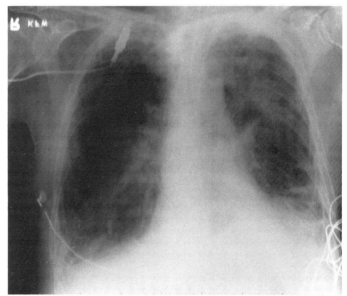

B

early interstitial pneumonitis, interstitial edema, and interstitial fibrosis.

The storage phosphor technology has been adapted to an AMBER type system to improve performance. It should be noted that the resolution of the storage phosphor is limited only by the precision of the laser scanning system that reads the latent image off the IP. Storage phosphor technology can rival traditional emulsion-based film detector systems in spatial resolution, with a contrast resolution or dynamic range which is much better than film.

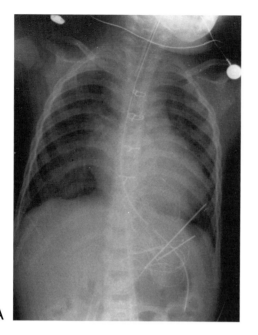 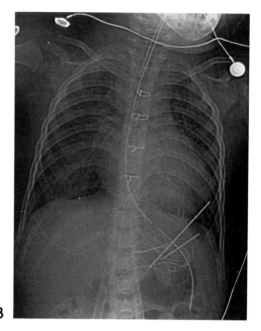

A   B

Fig. 2-11. **(A)** Pediatric chest image obtained with PSP detector and processed to produce a "conventional display." **(B)** Pediatric chest image obtained with PSP detector processed to enhance the visibility of the retrosternal and retrocardiac structures. Note increased conspicuity of endotracheal and nasotracheal tubes. Compare the cardiomegaly and the right lower lobe infiltrate in Figure 2-11A and B. (Courtesy of S. Balter, Ph.D.)

FILM DIGITIZATION

X-ray film can be used as the detector in a digital imaging system, in which case the film is subsequently digitized by using a microdensitometer or a video camera. This film digitization (FD) technique is a common method used in many simple teleradiology systems today. A wide latitude film can be used in an FD type system since the film is not used for viewing the image on the view box. Many experiments have been performed to examine the spatial resolution necessary to image diseases of the thorax by FD techniques.[17-19] The results of one of these studies has indicated that to evaluate mild interstitial lung disease and pneumothoraces the pixel size should be reduced to 0.1 mm × 0.1 mm,[17] which would correspond to a 4096 × 4096 × 10 bit image.

In another study using Dupont's Film Digital Radiography System (Film DRS), conventional radiographs and FD images were obtained for 150 patients.[18] The FD images, which had a spatial resolution of approximately 2.5 lp/mm, were viewed on a video monitor with interactive windowing capabilities. The video monitor displayed the images using a 1000 line system; the pixel size then was about 0.4 mm × 0.4 mm in the displayed digital images. There were 4096 gray levels, 12 bits, recorded and displayed. The Film DRS was used to digitize 100 abnormal and 50 normal conventional radiographs, obtained using various radiographic techniques, which were then viewed together with the nondigitized radiographs by four board-certified radiologists. The radiologists graded each of the radiographs on a scale of 1 to 10 for the presence

Fig. 2-12. **(A)** Pediatric chest image obtained with PSP detector and processed to produce a "conventional display." **(B)** Pediatric chest image obtained with PSP detector processed to enhance the visibility of the retrosternal and retrocardiac structures. Compare the appearance and visibility of the bilateral pneumothorax, and the right subcutaneous emphysema in Figures 2-12A and B. (Courtesy of S. Balter, Ph.D.)

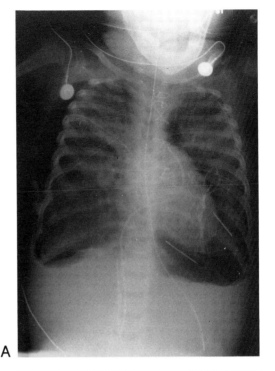

A

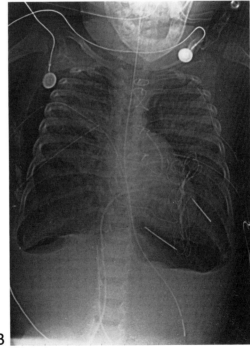

B

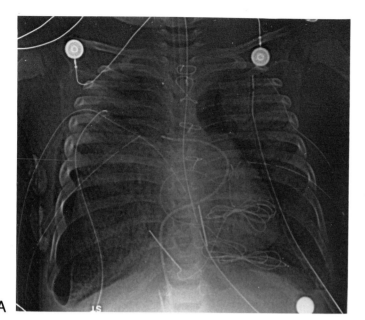

A

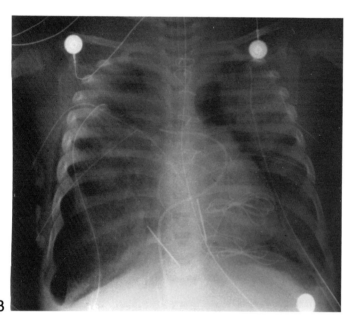

B

Fig. 2-13. (A) Pediatric chest image obtained with PSP detector and processed to produce a "conventional display." **(B)** Pediatric chest image obtained with PSP detector processed to enhance the visibility of the retrosternal and retrocardiac structures. Compare the appearance and visibility of the right pneumothorax and the right subcutaneous emphysema in Figures 2-13A and B. (Courtesy of S. Balter, Ph.D.)

of interstitial disease, pulmonary nodules, hilar and mediastinal disease, congestive heart failure, and hyperlucent conditions such as emphysema and pneumothorax. The results of this study indicated that the Film DRS system with interactive windowing was superior for the detection of hilar and mediastinal disease and that the conventional radiographs were better for the hyperlucent states. The two techniques were equivalent for the other categories. Digital radiography will continue to be a valuable technique in teleradiology systems; however, it is unlikely to be a practical substitute for DCR-type or AMBER systems.

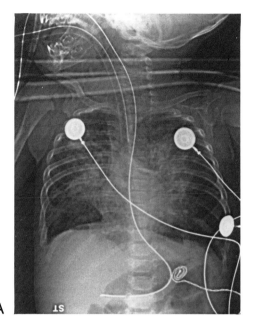

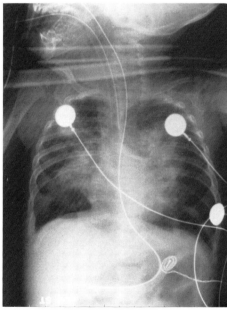

Fig. 2-14. (A) Digital pediatric chest image obtained using a PSP detector and processed to produce a conventional image appearance. **(B)** Digital pediatric chest image obtained using a PSP detector and processed to improve visibility of retrocardiac and retrosternal areas. Note increased conspicuity of endotracheal and nasotracheal tubes, and retrocardiac infiltrate in left lower lobe. (Courtesy of S. Balter, Ph.D.)

IMAGE INTENSIFIER

Digitizing the output from an image intensifier (II) has been very successful in digital subtraction angiography (DSA) (see Ch. 1). Application of this technology to the thorax has been limited both by the lack of a very large II capable of simultaneously imaging the entire thorax and by the limited spatial resolution of existing II systems. Recently, a system for chest imaging was reported[20] that is based on an II offering 33-, 40-, and 47-cm fields of view with a system resolution of 1.8 lp/mm. This system was shown to be equivalent to conventional radiography for the evaluation of pulmonary nodules. The II systems offer rapid dynamic imaging of the thorax but currently do not offer the spatial resolution to assess fine lung detail.

Pencil Beam Geometry

The one major limitation to traditional area beam x-ray detectors is the loss in image contrast that occurs because scattered radiation reaching the detector from the patient increases the signal to noise ratio. Conventional grids help in reducing the scattered radiation, but these are only partially successful.

The pencil beam detector system combines the use of a highly collimated x-ray beam, which is rapidly scanned across the entire chest in a raster-like fashion, with an x-ray detector. The detector, which may be a scintillation crystaltype, moves in synchrony with the x-ray beam behind the patient. Use of the pencil beam dramatically reduces the amount of scattered radiation reaching the detector. The exposure of the patient is extremely low. The positional information in the final image is derived from the relative x and y coordinates of the x-ray tube and detector as they are scanned over the area of interest. A prototype system was shown to have a resolution of 1.3 lp/mm with an exposure time of 5 seconds.[21] A pencil beam geometry system that was evaluated for detection of lung and mediastinal disease did not perform as well as conventional radiogra-

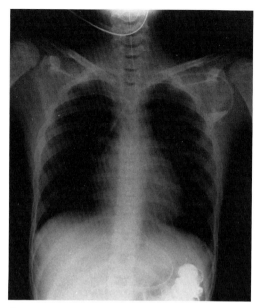

A

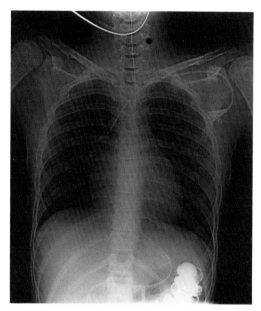

B

Fig. 2-15. (A) Digital PSP ICU chest image processed to display a conventional "film" appearance. **(B)** Digital ICU chest image processed to provide effective display of the entire chest including retrocardiac and retrosternal regions. (Courtesy of S. Balter, Ph.D.)

phy when an image matrix of 512 × 512 was used.[21] The pencil beam systems suffer from high x-ray tube heat loading and low spatial resolution.

Fan Beam Geometry

The newer SER and AMBER systems have good scatter rejection capability because of beam collimation and are more efficient than the pencil beam systems. Fan beam geometry utilizes scanning slits and scanning linear arrays of detectors to produce an image with less radiation scattering than DCR systems but less tube loading than a pencil beam system. A typical system will have a spatial resolution of 0.5 to 1.0 lp/mm. These scanning beam systems improve the detection of normal mediastinal anatomy and the detection of nodules overlying the mediastinum and diaphragm.[6] Dual energy detectors can be used with these systems, permitting acquisition of a high and a low energy image, which that can show soft tissue and bony detail, respectively. These dual energy systems can increase the conspicuity of a pulmonary nodule by subtracting out the bony structures of the thorax. They may also be used to assess the calcium content of pulmonary nodule.

ADVANTAGES OF DIGITAL SYSTEMS

Some digital imaging systems, including the systems with pencil beam and fan beam geometries, have superior scatter rejection as compared with DCR. The SER and AMBER systems also have improved scatter rejection, and it is presumed that these techniques will be incorporated into any new digital system.

Image processing is easily accomplished with digital systems because the image detector and display features are separated. The digital image can be processed by a variety of techniques and then displayed either by using a video display terminal or by writing the digital

Fig. 2-16. (A) Digital adult chest image processed to display a conventional "film" appearance. **(B)** Digital adult chest image processed to provide effective display of the entire chest including retrocardiac and retrosternal regions. (Courtesy of S. Balter, Ph.D.)

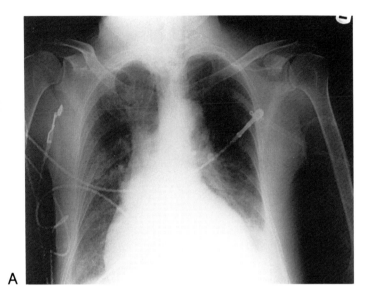

A

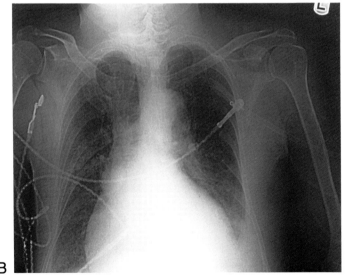

B

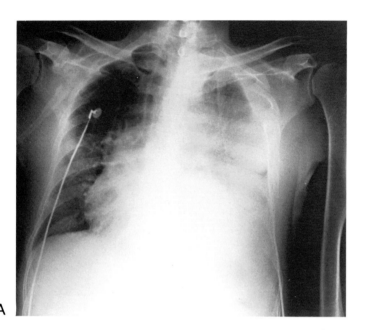

A

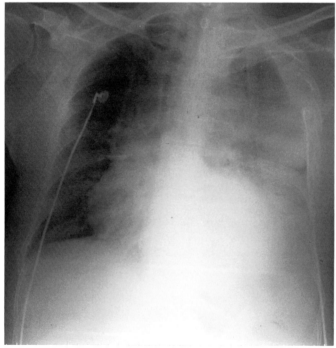

B

Fig. 2-17. (A) Digital adult chest image processed to display a conventional "film" appearance. **(B)** Digital adult chest image processed to provide effective display of the entire chest including retrocardiac and retrosternal regions. Compare the appearance and visibility of the left pleural effusion and the left pulmonary infiltrate in Figures 2-17A and B. (Courtesy of S. Balter, Ph.D.)

Fig. 2-18. (A) Digital adult chest image processed to display a conventional "film" appearance. **(B)** Digital adult chest image processed to provide effective display of the entire chest including retrocardiac and retrosternal regions. (Courtesy of S. Balter, Ph.D.)

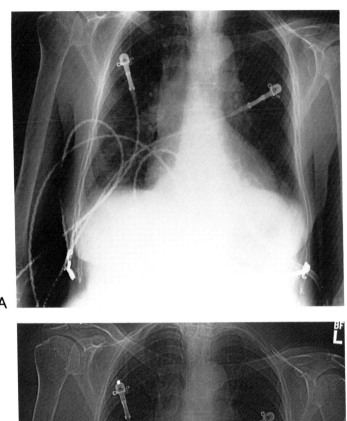

A

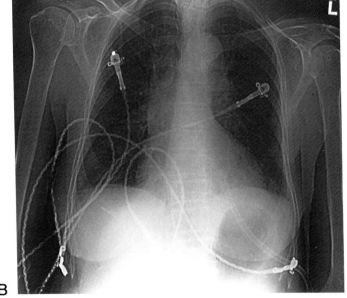

B

image back onto film using a laser camera. A number of image processing techniques have been applied to the processing of digital radiographs, including digital subtraction, high and low frequency filtration, histogram equalization, gray scale transformation, edge enhancement, unsharp masking, smoothing, and windowing and level control. Each processing technique emphasizes particular parts (edges, for example) of the final displayed image.

REFERENCES

1. Gray JE, Stears JF, Frank ED: Shaped, lead-loaded acrylic filters for patient exposure reduction and image-quality improvement. Radiology 146:825, 1983
2. Weder S, Adams PL: Improved routine chest radiography with a trough filter. AJR 137:695, 1981
3. Vyborny C, MacMahon H: Foil filters for equalized chest radiography. Radiology 151:154, 1984
4. Naimuddin S, Hasegawa BH, Dobbins JT, et al: Chest radiography using a digital beam attenuator. (Abstract). Radiology 153:38, 1984
5. Naimuddin S, Hasegawa BH, Dobins JT, et al: Selective exposure radiography of the chest. Med Phys 11:365, 1984
6. Goodman LR, Wilson CR, Foley WD: Digital radiography of the chest: Promises and problems. AJR 150:1241, 1988
7. Wandtke JC, Plewes DB, Vogelstein EE: Scanning equalization radiography of the chest: Assessment of image quality. AJR 145:973, 1985
8. Wandtke JC, Plewes DB, Vogelstein EE: Improved chest disease detection with scanning equalization radiography. AJR 145:979, 1985
9. Wandtke JC: Workshop: Newer techniques in chest radiography. Presented at Society of Thoracic Radiology Annual Meeting, San Diego, 1989
10. Niklason LT, Sorenson JA, Nelson JA: Scattered radiation in chest radiography. Med Phys 8:677, 1981
11. Vlasbloenm H, Kool LJSS: AMBER: A scanning multiple beam equalization system for chest radiography. Radiology 169:29, 1988
12. Seeley GW, Newell JD: The use of psychophysical principles in the design of a total digital radiology department. Radiol Clin North Am 23:341, 1985
13. Newell JD, Seeley G, Hagaman RM, et al: Computed radiographic evaluation of simulated pulmonary nodules—preliminary results. Invest Radiol 23:267, 1988
14. Fajardo LL, Hillman BJ, Pond GD: Detection of pneumothorax: Comparison of digital and conventional chest imaging. AJR 152:475, 1989
15. Furhman CR, Gur D, Good B, et al: Storage phosphor radiographs vs conventional films: Interpreter's perceptions of diagnostic quality. AJR 150:1011, 1988
16. Kangarloo H, Boechat MI, Barbaric Z, et al: Two-year clinical experience with a computed radiographic system. AJR 151:605, 1988
17. MacMahon H, Vyborny CJ, Metz CE, et al: Digital radiography of subtle pulmonary abnormalities: An ROC study of the effect of pixel size on observer performance. Radiology 158:21, 1986
18. Goodman LR, Foley WD, Wilson CR, et al: Digital and conventional chest images: Observer performance with film digital radiography system. Radiology 158:27, 1986
19. Lams PM, Cocklin ML: Spatial resolution requirements for digital chest radiographs: An ROC study of observer performance in selected cases. Radiology 158:11, 1986
20. Templeton AW, Dwyer SJ III, Cox GG, et al: A digital radiology imaging system: Description and clinical evaluation. AJR 149:847, 1987
21. Kushner DC, Cleveland RH, Herman TE, et al: Low-dose flying spot digital radiography of the chest: Sensitivity studies. Radiology 163:685, 1987

3

Digital Genitourinary, Gastrointestinal, and Breast Radiology

Tim B. Hunter
Laurie L. Fajardo

INTRODUCTION

Computer-assisted imaging was successfully introduced into diagnostic radiology in the 1970s. The need for computers resulted from the complex mathematical reconstructions that are required to perform nuclear medicine, computed tomography (CT), and ultrasound examinations. More recently, digital subtraction angiography (DSA) and magnetic resonance imaging (MRI) have further amplified the importance of digital technology to diagnostic imaging.

While digital techniques are thus well established in some areas of diagnostic radiology, they have made little impact in genitourinary (GU), gastrointestinal (GI), and breast

imaging. Traditional screen-film GU, GI, and mammography studies produce excellent diagnostic information at reasonable cost and are the best methods available at this time. However, digital imaging has several inherent advantages over everyday screen-film analog techniques, including lower radiation dose, wider image latitude, and image processing capability. These advantages will become increasingly important in the future. This chapter explores a variety of miscellaneous areas in which digital techniques may be useful but not yet established. We hope to point out prime topics for research as well as to discuss the present diagnostic capabilities of digital imaging for the GI and GU systems and for the breast.

THE COMPUTED RADIOGRAPHIC SYSTEM: TECHNICAL CONSIDERATIONS

A photostimulated phosphor (PSP)-based computed radiography system consists of several components (Fig. 3-1). The x-ray receptor is an imaging plate composed of a plastic substrate containing europium-doped barium fluorohalide crystals, which are photostimulable.[1,2] These crystals can be raised to a higher energy state by exposure to x-rays and can store this energy for later release when the imaging plate is read by the system's scanning laser. The imaging plate has a linear dynamic range of 10,000:1, approximately 10 times that of conventional screen-film combinations. Its spatial resolution is 2.5 to 5 line pairs per millimeter (lp/mm), depending upon the size and type (standard or high resolution) of imaging plate used. A far greater range of exposures can be accommodated with a computed radiography system than with a conventional screen-film system, and the imaging plates are reusable, lasting for more than 8,000 exposures.

Image Formation

After exposure, the imaging plate is scanned by a low-power laser beam (exposure data recognizer) to determine both the overall exposure and the dynamic range of tissues to be visualized. The imaging plate is then rescanned with a high intensity helium-neon laser beam, and the resultant energy, released as blue phosphorescence, is conducted via a light pipe to a photomultiplier tube for conversion into an electrical signal. These electronic signals are digitized into 10 bits or 1,024 gray levels. The 10 bits are fully utilized regardless of the radiation exposure used to form the image. This means that the specific densities of interest (e.g., soft tissues, pararenal fat, calculi, iodinated contrast media, etc.) have

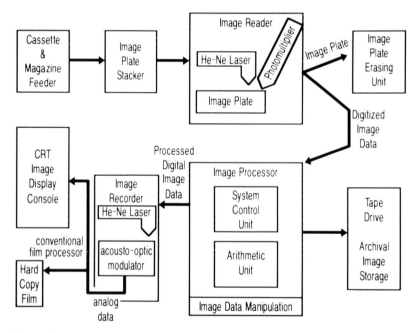

Fig. 3-1. The Toshiba computed radiography TCR 201 system. (Courtesy of Toshiba Medical Systems, Tustin, CA.)

their relative specific absorption characteristics expanded or contracted to fit the H and D response curve of the film used for display. The digital information is transferred to a central processing unit and stored.

After processing, the digitized image is passed through a digital-to-analog (D/A) converter. The resultant analog signals modulate the intensity of another helium-neon laser beam by means of an acousto-optical modulator.[3] The modulated laser beam "paints" each line of the image onto a single emulsion film, which can be used for a hard copy. Images can also be displayed on a cathode-ray tube (CRT) console (512×512 matrix).

Image Enhancement for Excretory Urography

Performing GU radiographic imaging by computed radiography allows post-processing of image data, which is accomplished primarily by two user-controlled functions, frequency processing and gradation processing. Frequency processing affects the sharpness of an image by creating a blurred subtraction image from the original. The frequency response of the resultant image is enhanced over a range selected by the observer to a degree that depends on the signal strength at a particular point on the image. For observing fine detail such as bony ridges, high frequency processing is used; for evaluating large patterns such as the kidneys, low frequency processing is used. When performing computed excretory urography, it is often advantageous to produce a pair of images for each exposure. One image is processed by an algorithm that simulates a conventional radiograph with use of a nonlinear gradient curve and a maximum spatial frequency of about 0.25 cycles per millimeter (Fig. 3-2, right). The second image in the pair is a frequency-modified image (Fig. 3-2, left) that is produced with a nonlinear gradient and sixfold enhancement of normal spatial frequency. This process enhances the edges of structures and increases the conspicuity of

dense objects such as stones (Fig. 3-3), foreign bodies (Fig. 3-4), and some mass-kidney interfaces (Fig. 3-5).

The final step in image production, gradation processing, changes the relationship between optical density and input, rather as if one could choose from many different films, each with its own characteristic H and D curve. In addition to selecting from a range of contrast relationships, an input-density curve can be shifted along the input signal axis. This changes the relationships of signal input to density, making the film lighter or darker (Fig. 3-6). It is also possible to rotate the data around a selected point on the curve, which primarily affects the resultant contrast of the image; a steeper angle provides for a shorter contrast scale, while a slowly rising curve allows for a broader contrast range (Fig. 3-7). These manipulations have potential for evaluating particularly dark or light areas of the image for suspected abnormalities. Because the image data are easily retrieved, the net effect of these operations is equivalent to providing the user with a limitless number of different output films, each with its own speed and contrast characteristics to enhance diagnostic detail.

GENITOURINARY RADIOLOGY

Digital technology has recently been very successfully applied to GU tract imaging. Advantages of computed radiography in this field include a wide dynamic range of acceptable exposures as compared with conventional screen-film combinations plus the ability to selectively match the computed radiography system's response characteristics to a specific radiographic examination. There is also a significant reduction in radiation exposure. These features improve radiographic diagnosis, reduce radiation dose to patients, and have the potential to decrease operating cost.

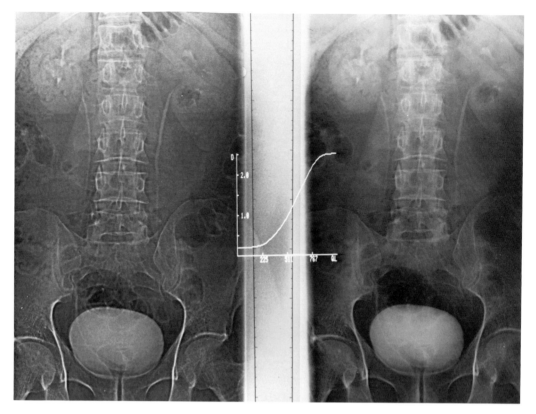

Fig. 3-2. Typical digital image pair produced from a single urographic exposure. The image on the right is processed with an algorithm simulating a conventional radiograph. The left image is a frequency-modified (edge-enhanced) image. (QL = output image signal [frequency processed signal]; D = output density.)

Clinical Genitourinary Applications of Digital Imaging

We have recently completed the evaluation of 100 excretory urograms by using paired digital and screen-film examinations.[4,5] There was no statistical difference in diagnostic efficacy between the two modalities. Particularly noteworthy is that edge-enhanced digital images demonstrated cortical scarring and ureteral calculi more prominently than did screen-film radiographs. When radiologists rated the quality of digital urographic images compared with screen-film images, no difference was found, which provides further evidence that digital technology is suitable for use in urography.[6,7]

We have also evaluated patients before and after extracorporeal shock wave lithotripsy and found better depiction of stone fragments on edge-enhanced digital tomograms.[8]

We performed digital urography at an average radiation dose of 53 percent of that used for screen-film urography. The ability to produce images at lower radiation doses is especially helpful when it is necessary to examine pregnant women. A three- to four-image digital urogram can be obtained at the same exposure dose used for a single abdominal radiograph by conventional screen-film methods. We have also obtained diagnostically useful

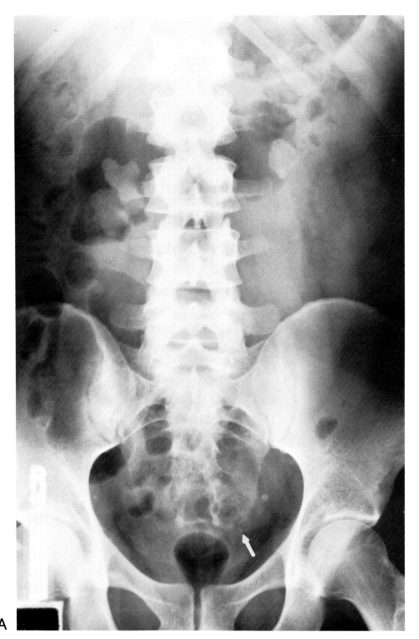

Fig. 3-3. (**A**) Film-screen radiograph. *(Figure continues.)*

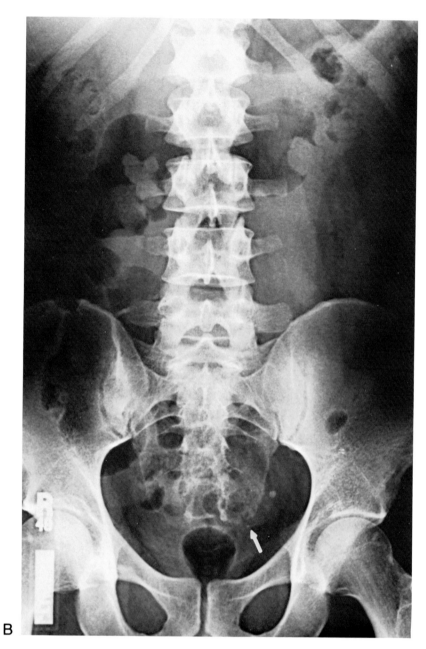

B

Fig. 3-3 *(Continued).* **(B & C)** Digital image pair demonstrating distal left ureteral calculus (arrow). *(Figure continues.)*

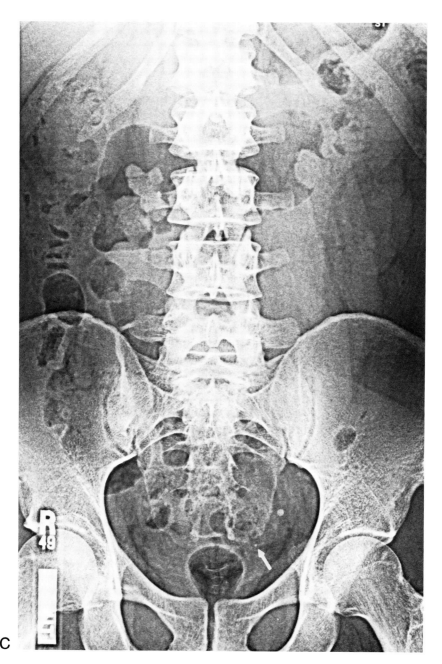

C

Fig. 3-3 (*Continued*). **(C)** Although visible on the film-screen image, the calculus is best appreciated on the edge-enhanced digital image radiograph.

images at 25 to 33 percent of the usual radiation dose for determination of fetal position prior to delivery (Fig. 3-8).

GASTROINTESTINAL RADIOLOGY

Because imaging plate techniques offer a wider exposure latitude (system dynamic range) than screen-film techniques, patient dose can often be reduced and poor radiographic technique partially alleviated by postprocessing. That is, "films" that are too dark or too light may be adjusted to obtain diagnostic images. This is particularly advantageous for portable chest, abdomen, and extremity work, where poor technique and unpredictable output from the portable equipment are constant problems. In addition, the digital images have the potential for further improvement by edge, contrast, and brightness enhancement.

Pond and his co-workers, in a prospective study comparing digital photostimulable imaging plate radiography with conventional screen-film radiography in 26 patients undergoing intraoperative arteriography and in 40 patients undergoing operative or endoscopic cholangiography, found the radiation dose to be reduced by 50 percent with the digital imaging plate technique.[9] No repeat digital arteriograms or cholangiograms were required, while 5 percent of the screen-film studies had to be repeated owing to under- or overexposure. The imaging plate studies did require slightly more time for processing (an average of 35 seconds per patient). Receiver operating characteristic (ROC) analysis showed no significant difference in the diagnostic accuracy between the two competing imaging techniques for either the arteriographic or the cholangiographic studies. Observer preference was the same for the screen-film and the digital techniques.

In this study by Pond et al., the digital imaging plate technique was also found to be satisfactory for evaluation of newly placed or revised arterial bypass grafts and hemodialysis fistulae. Digital imaging was also successful in a wide range of cholangiographic applications, including operative cholangiography following cholecystectomy, and in routine endoscopic retrograde cholangiopancreatography (Fig. 3-9). Adequate diagnoses were made of residual arterial thrombi; distal emboli; intimal flaps; anastomotic stenoses, including bile duct stenoses; arteriovenous fistulae; retained bile duct calculi; contrast extravasation from vessels or the biliary system; and adequacy of biliary bypass.

Digital imaging techniques are particularly applicable for operating room and portable radiography. Surgeons doing contrast injections during angiography and cholangiography often cannot wear lead aprons because of the sterile conditions mandatory in the operating theater. To keep radiation levels to a minimum, scout films for setting up proper technique are usually omitted, and therefore it is most important to obtain adequate studies from the very first exposure. Digital processing greatly aids this effort because "light" or "dark" images can be corrected while at the same time there is general reduction in radiation levels. Obviating repeat exposures not only decreases the radiation level for the patient and operating room personnel but also reduces the anesthesia time. Similar considerations apply to portable radiographs obtained on the wards or in intensive care units. Repeat examinations are discomforting for the patient and greatly inconvenience the nursing personnel and radiology technicians involved. Moreover, digital radiology has the added advantage of possible widespread distribution of the images over a local area network so that the referring physicians and radiologists can view the studies at remote locations.

Most digitized radiographs and all digital imaging plate examinations suffer from the distinct disadvantage of reduced spatial resolution compared with routine screen-film radiographs. The typical resolution of present digi-

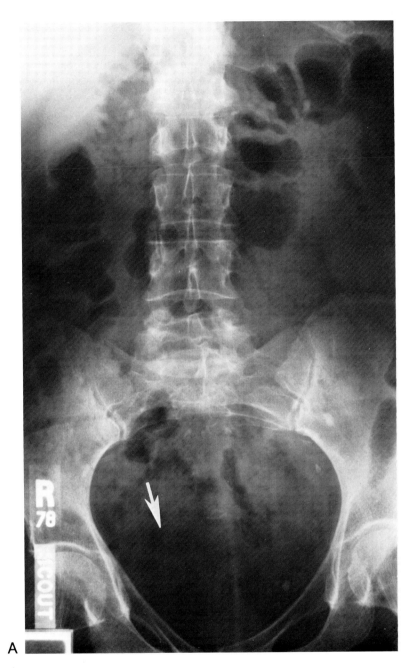

Fig. 3-4. **(A)** Conventional screen-film abdominal image. *(Figure continues.)*

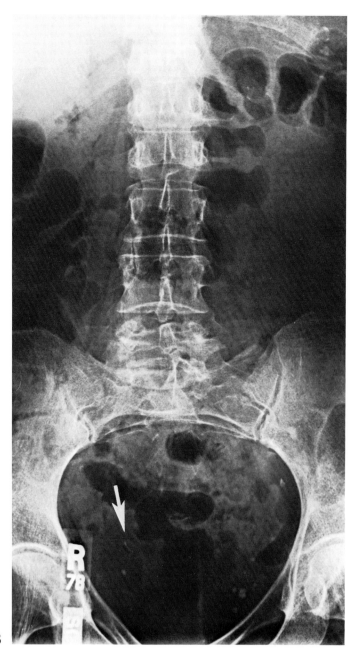

B

Fig. 3-4 *(Continued).* **(B & C)** Digital abdominal images demonstrating retained surgical needle (arrow), which was diagnosed only on the digital study. Note increased conspicuity due to edge enhancement in Figure C. *(Figure continues.)*

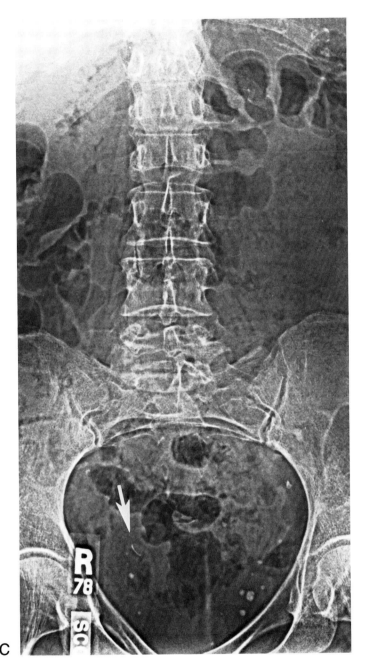

Fig. 3-4 *(Continued).*

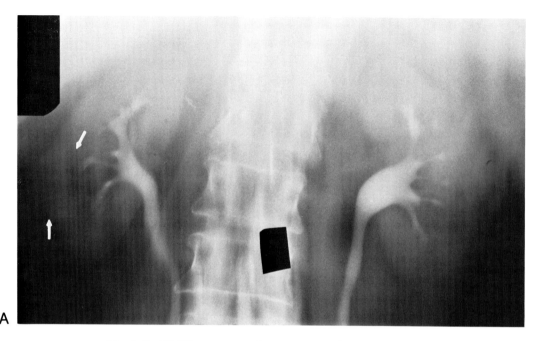

Fig. 3-5. (A) Film-screen nephrotomogram. *(Figure continues.)*

tal systems is 2.5 lp/mm vs. at least 5 lp/mm for conventional studies. Unfortunately, there is no consensus as to the needed spatial resolution for a given type of diagnostic examination. Preliminary work at the University of Arizona suggests that a resolution of 2.5 lp/mm is sufficient for vascular, cholangiographic, urographic, and barium GI studies. Higher spatial resolutions may certainly be necessary for bone, chest, or mammographic examinations. In general, digital imaging greatly enhances contrast resolution at the expense of spatial resolution. Improved contrast resolution, to a certain extent, can overcome loss of spatial detail, but the trade-off between these two parameters for a particular application remains largely unknown.[10-15]

Another disadvantage of present digital imaging systems is that they often write the final image onto a relatively small film format. Radiologists, and especially referring physicians, frequently object to chest and abdominal images on a format of 8 × 10 inches instead of the familiar format of at least 10 × 12 inches or, more usually, 14 × 17 inches.[12] This reluctance can be hard to overcome, and we have had referring physicians refuse to accept digital imaging studies for their patients. Larger formats in the near future will help, as will increasing physician familiarity with nonstandard film imaging.

Digital workstations with high resolution CRTs are in active use in many departments and are readily accepted. We have encountered one interesting problem that has not been commented upon by others. The cooling fans and other moving parts in some of the prototype digital workstations have very high noise levels. The noise is quite annoying and unacceptable for long-term use and could conceivably cause some hearing impairment if one were subjected to it for months or years. Obviously, this noise can be controlled by acoustic shielding of equipment and separation of the computing portion of the digital workstation from the viewing screens. Another, most

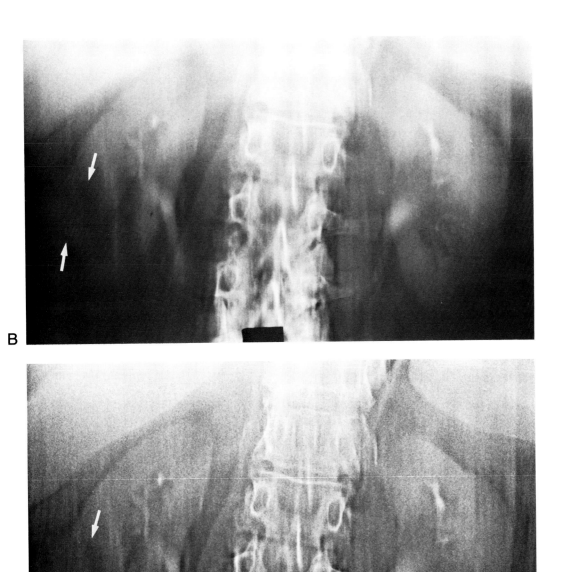

Fig. 3-5 *(Continued).* **(B & C)** Digital nephrotomograms demonstrating right lower pole renal mass (arrows).

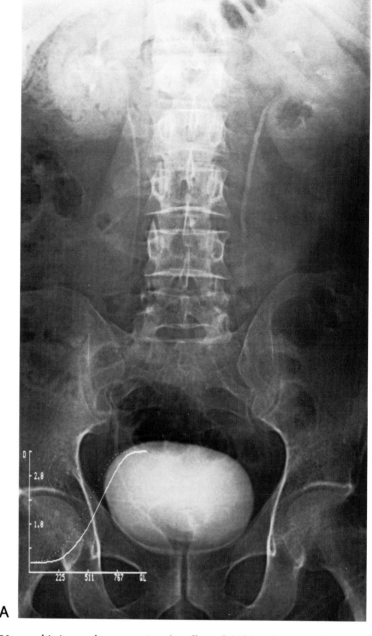

A

Fig. 3-6. (A) Urographic image demonstrating the effect of shifting the input-density curve toward the left. *(Figure continues.)*

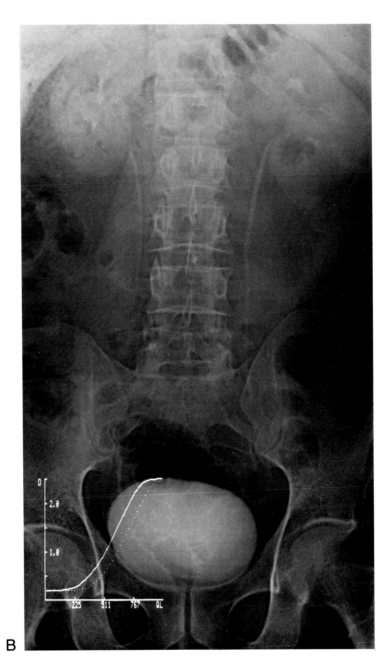

B

Fig. 3-6 *(Continued).* **(B)** Urographic image demonstrating the effect of shifting the input-density curve toward the right. The solid curve corresponds to the input-density curve used for urographic scout abdominal and compression-release films, as illustrated in Figure 3-2. (QL = frequency-processed output image signal; D = output density.)

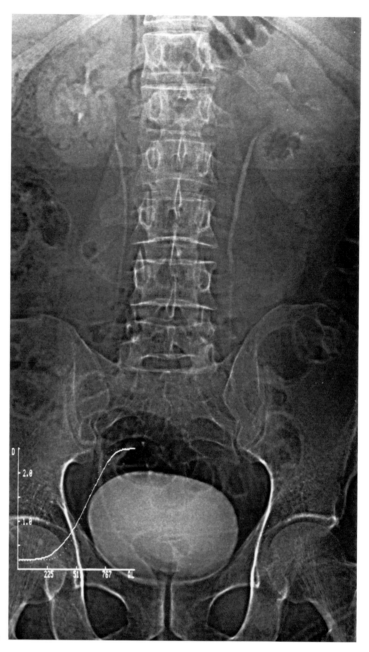

Fig. 3-7. Effects of rotating the input-density curve about a specific point (D = 1.2). Varying the degree of rotation to **(A)** a lesser slope narrows the contrast scale. *(Figure continues.)*

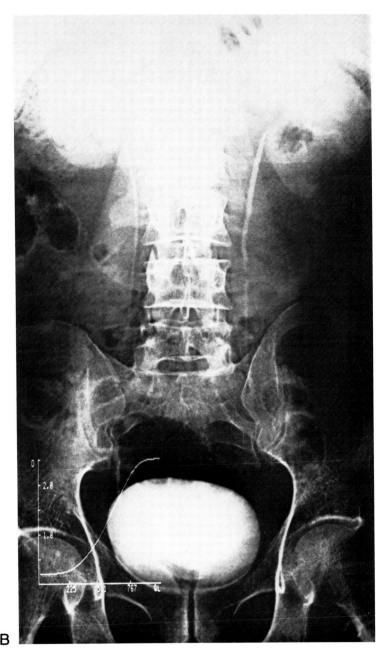

B

Fig. 3-7 *(Continued).* **(B)** A greater rotation alters the slope of the resultant input-density curve broadening the contrast scale. (Solid curve is density curve for images in Fig. 3-2).

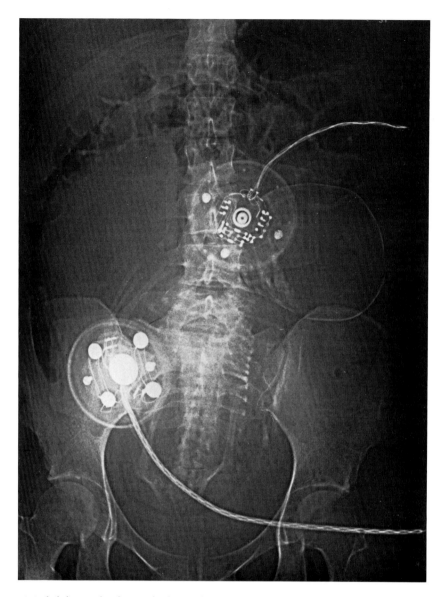

Fig. 3-8. Digital abdominal radiograph obtained to evaluate fetal position (frank breech). The image was produced with a 75 percent reduction in the usual radiation dose used with conventional screen-film radiography.

important consideration in the production and transmission of digital images from one location or device to another is whether the applicable devices conform to standards set by the American College of Radiology and National Electrical Manufacturers Association (ACR-NEMA 300-1985). These standards are now well defined and are being actively promoted so that devices and software from different manufacturers have certain levels of compatibility.

There has been less formal investigation of the applicability of digital imaging for routine barium GI studies than for DSA and GU stud-

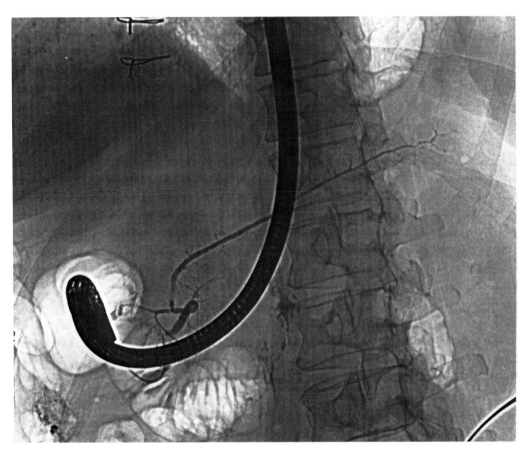

Fig. 3-9. Endoscopic retrograde cholangiopancreatography performed with the Toshiba TCR 201 system. A normal main pancreatic duct is readily evident.

ies. Anecdotal experience at the University of Arizona with the Toshiba Computed Radiology (TCR) system shows that the quality of upper GI series, barium enemas (Fig. 3-10A & B) and enteroclysis studies (Fig. 3-10C & D), is approximately the same as with conventional screen-film examinations. There appears to be enough spatial resolution for accurate diagnosis, but there is a definite time disadvantage with the present system. It takes several minutes for the final overhead or spot film images to become available for viewing either on film or on a high resolution monitor. This is a problem with GI studies. Often the radiologist cannot afford to wait long for a particular image, especially if the patient's colon is full of barium!

The enhanced contrast resolution available with digital imaging is less of an advantage for barium and water-soluble iodine examinations, as these techniques already provide inherently high contrast. Because of this and because of the long processing times for the images, acceptance of digital radiology for everyday barium studies has been slow. Nevertheless, digital imaging for traditional GI work and plain abdominal films will pose no major problems when equipment giving a more rapid turnaround becomes available. Even now, 13 percent of all the computed radiography system images on the University of California at Los Angeles digital system are for plain abdominal radiographic examinations, and these are obtained with a 33 percent re-

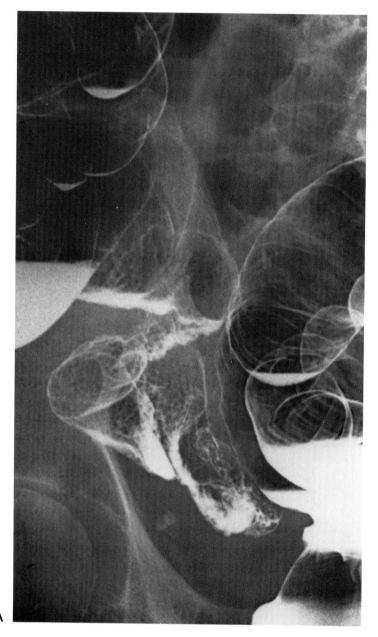

Fig. 3-10. (A & B) Air-contrast barium enemas performed with the Toshiba TCR 201. Figure A shows Crohn's disease in the terminal ileum. *(Figure continues.)*

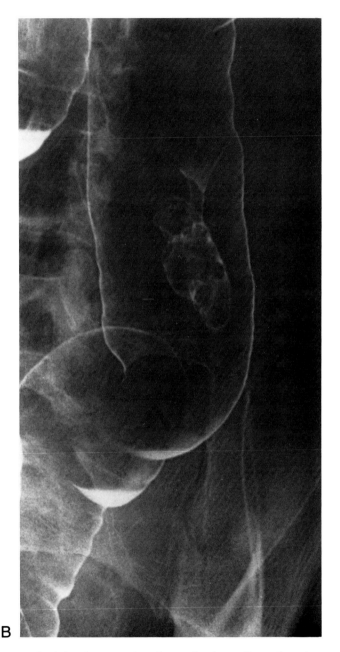

B

Fig. 3-10 *(Continued).* **(B)** A large sessile polyp in the descending colon. *(Figure continues.)*

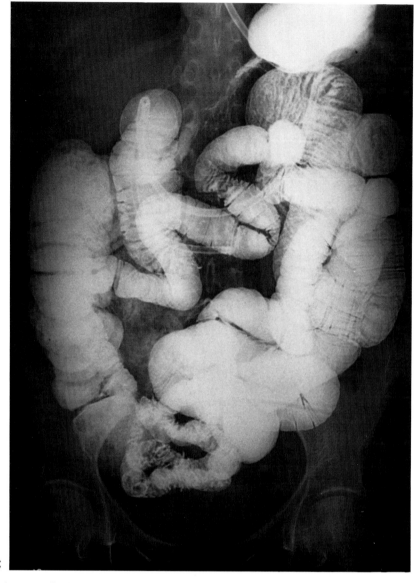

C

Fig. 3-10 *(Continued).* **(C)** Enteroclysis study performed with the Toshiba TCR 201. *(Figure continues.)*

duction in dose to the average pediatric patient.[12]

Children are the only class of patients who routinely receive a lower dose following a switch to a digital system. If it were possible to reduce the dose without excessive image quality degradation, faster screen-film contributions would be used. Many pediatric patients are so small that a certain minimal dose is re-

quired to lift the screen-film response out of the "toe" region of the characteristic curve. Digital systems do not have a toe region and hence can form acceptable images in pediatric patients at lower doses.

Our own experience has also been that the TCR system is excellent for a variety of plain film applications. Abdominal studies with portable equipment to locate the position of feed-

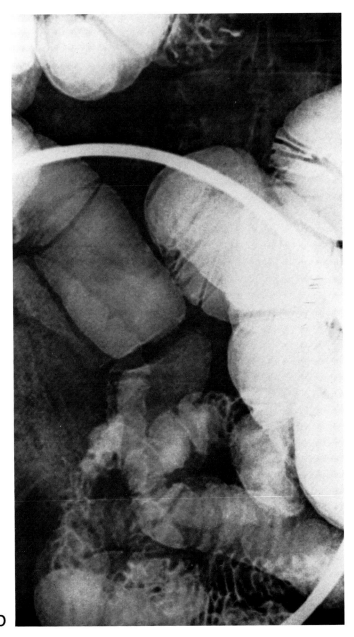

Fig. 3-10 *(Continued)*. **(D)** A coned view of a subtle narrowing caused by a small bowel adhesion.

ing tubes and nasogastric tubes are routinely performed by computed radiography because of lower patient dose and a greatly reduced examination repeat rate. Renal and biliary calculi are readily seen and bowel obstruction is readily diagnosed. Physician acceptance over conventional plain film studies is especially good where tubes, calculi, or foreign bodies are being sought, but it is somewhat poor in those instances in which subtle bowel obstruction may be present or sinus tract injections are being performed. This stems in part from the generally smaller image format size with computed radiography and in part from the slow turnaround times for a dynamic study; as with sinus tract injections. Younger physicians less accustomed to the more traditional examinations seem more willing to accept the newer imaging modalities. On the other hand, the conventional screen-film barium techniques will be in use for many years to come. They are familiar, relatively inexpensive, and produce great diagnostic accuracy with rapid patient throughput. The present computed radiographic techniques, while important for the future, are not acceptable yet for the everyday busy GI radiology suite.

Routine digital fluoroscopy, as opposed to portable c-arm digital fluoroscopy or to the use of computed imaging plate radiography for overhead and spot films, is not yet available or practical for most departments. Cost considerations—along with severe limitations on image size, image acquisition speeds, and image storage—are the main problems. Because computer memory is inadequate for archival storage of images, the memory is used to contain pictures only while they are being processed. Magnetic hard disc drives are then used for intermediate storage, with archiving onto optical laser discs for long-term storage. Disc speed itself limits the speed of image acquisition and, additionally, if there is image digitization with high bit levels,[10-12] the storage capacity of a disc system may be quite limiting. Fortunately, fast digital disc systems are available; for example, present DSA systems acquire and store four or more image frames per second. If there is ultrarapid image acquisition (20 to 30 images per second), the pictures are stored in main memory and then transferred to the disc drive during periods of lower use.

A major unsolved problem is how to handle the long-term storage and retrieval of multiple GI images for a large number of patient examinations. This is especially true if there are several minutes of fluoroscopy for each patient. At 30 frames per second (to avoid flicker) and at a spatial resolution of 1024×1024 pixels

with 8 to 10 gray levels, the storage capacity needed becomes astronomical, and data compression becomes an absolute necessity. Interestingly, it is uncertain how fast fluoroscopic images need to be acquired and displayed. Viewing speeds of less than 15 to 30 frames per second cause visible image flicker, which may be upsetting to the observer. On the other hand, an observer may accept the display of only a few images per second. This gives a reasonable pseudo-real-time effect and may be acceptable for gastrointestinal diagnosis. These considerations require much further research before we can expect widespread introduction of fully digital fluoroscopic systems.

Another area promising some applicability for GI diagnosis but requiring considerable research is that of dual energy subtraction techniques. Several different approaches have been taken. One approach was by Hunter et al., who generated quasimonochromatic beams by the filtration of conventional x-ray sources, thereby producing x-ray spectra on the low and high energy sides of the contrast element absorption edge.[16] If one beam is centered at Ef_1 40 keV and another beam is centered at Ef_2 90 keV and if two exposures are taken at Ef_1 and Ef_2 in rapid succession followed by subtraction of the quasimonochromatic images, inhaled xenon gas can be used to produce excellent radiographic opacification of the tracheal airway. In addition, superb visualization of the gallbladder and bile ducts in normal volunteers may be seen with one-fourth to one-half the usual dose of Oragrafin Calcium (Fig. 3-11). These techniques, coupled with high band pass filtering and edge enhancement, may have some future applicability in biliary duct, gallbladder, airway, and bowel imaging.

BREAST RADIOLOGY

Mammography is the "gold standard" for breast diagnosis. It is a widely accepted fact that more breast malignancies are diagnosed by mammography than by physical examina-

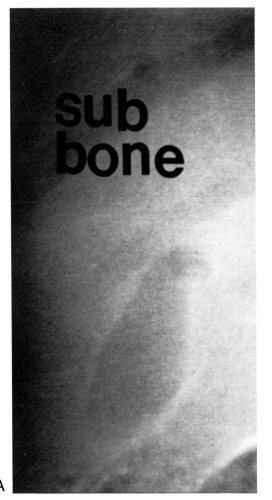 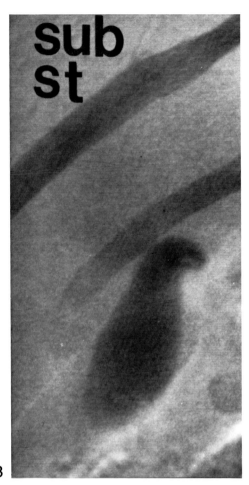

A   B

Fig. 3-11. Digital dual energy subtraction study of the gallbladder. A normal volunteer was given one-fourth the usual dose of Oragrafin Calcium. Processing is shown for **(A)** bone subtraction and **(B)** soft tissue subtraction.

tion, breast sonography, or light scanning. Nonetheless, these procedures are complementary rather than competitive because a significant proportion (5 to 15 percent) of all breast cancers are overlooked on mammography and detected by other means, principally breast physical examination. However, mammography is often capable of detecting tiny lesions before they enlarge enough to become palpable and at a stage at which they apparently have not metastasized and are curable.

Small calcifications are one of the earliest and most reliable, although nonspecific, findings of in situ and early, minimally invasive breast cancer. Detection of such lesions truly tests the ability of present digital systems, all of which have a far lower spatial resolution than conventional screen-film systems.[17,18] Even digitization of conventional mammographic films with a fine 0.1 × 0.1 mm pixel size degrades the detectability of microcalcifications. In preliminary work on a breast phantom study, Oestmann and colleagues found that the TCR 201 digital mammography system localized the same number of calcification clusters as conventional screen-film mammography but could not distinguish individual calcifications as well.[18] For this experiment the storage phosphor imaging plates were laser-scanned, with a 100-μm sampling pitch. The images had a 2000 × 2510 pixel matrix with 10 bits of gray levels. The effective resolution of the digital images was 6 lp/mm vs. a nominal 15 lp/mm for conventional screen-film mammography.

The mere ability to detect breast calcification clusters, without the ability to evaluate their individual microcalcifications well, may be insufficient for clinical use. Further, systematic imaging studies, with a wide variety of in vitro materials followed by prospective clinical trials, are necessary to properly determine the diagnostic capabilities of digital imaging. Future development of higher resolution systems would naturally obviate the disadvantages of the present systems. Unfortunately, the 10 lp/mm and higher resolutions needed to approximate the screen-film resolution appear to be a considerable distance in the future because of severe technical problems. Such high resolution systems would further aggravate the already familiar problems with picture archiving and communication systems of how to store, retrieve, and transmit large numbers of high resolution pictures.

Even given the above considerations, digital breast imaging may have an important ancillary role along with routine mammography. It might be used for screening and transmission of images on large numbers of patients, with screen-film views being reserved for suspicious areas. It might also be used when the number of film retakes caused by over- or underexposure needs to be reduced. Digital imaging could even help to detect large low-contrast masses hidden by surrounding dense breast tissue. It is certain that digital breast imaging will become more important in the early 1990s, but its role may remain secondary to that of traditional mammography well into the middle of the decade.

Up to the present (1990), digital breast studies have been accomplished by digitization of screen-film images or by production of images on laser-scanned storage phosphor systems such as the Toshiba TCR 201. Fluoroscopy with real-time imaging of breast tissue is an intriguing idea but not practical, owing to the low kilovoltage necessary for poor contrast breast tissues. A new type of imaging receptor is needed. Along these lines, one very exciting area for research is the use of charge-coupled devices (CCDs), which are small chips (about 1 cm square) that are extraordinarily sensitive to visible light. They have virtually no lag, and each pixel element can act as an individual radiation detector. Their light sensitivity and electronic characteristics are such that they have almost completely replaced film photography in professional astronomy.

We, as well as other groups, are now investigating the use of CCDs in diagnostic radiology. They lack a large field area and are relatively insensitive to x-rays but can detect more photons emitted by an intensifying screen than can radiographic film. Because of their small size, they must be optically coupled to the intensifier screen either through a lens arrangement or through the use of optic fibers. This allows the viewing of only a small body area, perhaps 4 to 6 inches square. Because of their limited size and resolution (about 1000 × 1000 to 2000 × 2000 pixel elements for expensive CCDs), CCDs cannot presently be used for routine mammography. However, they have extremely high speed and can produce an image on a CRT screen in 1 second or less when linked to appropriate hardware and software.

Present experimentation uses a system in which a breast phantom is radiographed by a routine mammography unit. The x-rays pass through the phantom or patient breast and strike a high efficiency mammography screen.

The light from the screen is then optically fed to the CCD system, which displays the image on a CRT screen in 1 second or less. Preliminary work has shown that the sensitivity of such an arrangement is at least as good as that of the fastest mammography screen-film combinations. With the use of high efficiency CCDs and optical fiber coupling to an optimally designed intensifying screen, it would be possible to reduce the present patient exposures by at least a factor of 10!

CCD technology offers the possibility for pseudo-real-time mammography, in which mammography images are taken and displayed as fast as x-ray tube exposure times and heat dissipation allow. Needle localization or lesion biopsy would be much easier with a CCD biplane unit, optimized for x-ray tube output and speed and CCD resolution and size. In the mid-1990s routine mammography might be performed with a standard screen-film setup, after which any suspicious lesions could be immediately biopsied with CCD mammography equipment. The practitioner would actually watch the biopsy needle go into the area of interest with real-time imaging. With improvement in CCD technology and cost, all breast imaging could eventually be performed with CCDs exclusively. CCD images have exquisite contrast resolution and all the advantages of other digital images. Some day radiologists may sit in their offices monitoring breast examinations on a remote display as they are being obtained. When suspicious lesions are seen, they could then walk down to the mammography suite and perform a real-time biopsy before the patient leaves the department. This concept is only a dream but is theoretically possible with 1980s technology. It may become a working reality for the 1990s with the CCD and mammography system technology.

REFERENCES

1. Leverenz HW: An Introduction to Luminescences of Solids. Dover Publications, New York, 1968

2. Arnold BA, Eisenberg H, Boyer D, Metherell A: Digital radiography: An overview. SPIE Vol 273. Application of Optical Instruments for Medicine 9:215, 1981

3. Sonoda M, Takano M, Miyahara J, Kato H: Computed radiography utilizing scanning laser stimulated luminescence. Radiology 148:833, 1983

4. Fajardo LL, Hillman BJ, Hunter TB, et al: Prospective comparison of digital and screen-film urography — 100 patients. Radiological Society of North America, 72nd Scientific Assembly, Chicago, Nov. 30 — Dec. 5, 1986

5. Fajardo LL, Hillman BJ, Hunter TB, et al: Excretory urography using a computed radiography system. Radiology 162:345, 1987

6. Fajardo LL, Hillman BJ: Correlations among image quality, radiologists' certainty of diagnosis, and accuracy in interpreting digital and screen-film urograms. Association of University Radiologists, 35th Annual Meeting, Charleston, SC, Mar. 22–27, 1987

7. Fajardo LL, Hillman BJ: Image quality, diagnostic certainty, and accuracy: Comparison of conventional and digital urograms. Urol Radiol 10(3):21, 1988

8. Sacks EM, Hillman BJ, Fajardo LL, et al: Evaluation of ESWL results by conventional and digital tomography. Radiologic Society of North America, 73rd Scientific Assembly, Chicago, Nov. 29–Dec. 4, 1987

9. Pond GD, Seeley GW, Yoshino MT, et al: Comparison of conventional screen-film to photostimulable imaging plate radiographs for intraoperative arteriography and cholangiography. SPIE Vol. 914. Medical Imaging 11:139, 1988

10. Swets JA, Pickett RM: Evaluation of Diagnostic Systems. Academic Press, Orlando, FL, 1982

11. Gould RG: Digital hardware in radiography and fluoroscopy. Appl Radiol 13:137, 1984

12. Kangarloo H, Boechat MI, Barbaric Z, et al: Two year clinical experience with a computed radiography system. AJR 151:605, 1988

13. Merritt CRB, Tutton RH, Bell KA, et al: Clinical application of digital radiography: Computed radiographic imaging. Radiographics 5:397, 1985

14. Tateno Y, Iinuma T, Takano M (eds): Computed Radiography. Springer-Verlag, New York, 1987

15. Huang HK: Elements of Digital Radiography. Prentice-Hall, Englewood Cliffs, NJ, 1987

16. Hunter TB, Pond GB, Roehrig H: Gastrointestinal radiology using dual energy imaging. (Abstract). 31st Annual Meeting, Association of University Radiologists, Mar. 22–25, Mobile, AL, 1983

17. Chan HP, Vyborny CJ, MacMahon H, et al: Digital mammography: ROC studies of the effect of pixel size and unsharp-mask filtering on the detection of subtle microcalcifications. Invest Radiol 22:581, 1987

18. Oestmann JW, Kopans D, Hall DA, et al: A comparison of digitized storage phosphors and conventional mammography in the detection of malignant microcalcifications. Invest Radiol 23:725, 1988

4

Teleradiology

John D. Newell, Jr.

INTRODUCTION

Teleradiology is the transmission and interpretation of radiologic images at a site remote from that at which the images were acquired. It can use many modern digital imaging and digital telecommunication techniques. In this chapter the history of teleradiology and the fundamental elements of a practical digital teleradiology system are examined, and the experience obtained by several investigators studying digital teleradiology systems is discussed. The practical advantages of a phone-based digital teleradiology system are emphasized, together with the shortcomings of such a system. The prospect for developing faster phone-based digital teleradiology techniques is also examined.

HISTORICAL BACKGROUND

In 1959 Dr. Albert Jutra linked two hospitals in Montreal by using teleradiology techniques.[1,2] The 5-mile distance between the hospitals was spanned with coaxial cable,

which transmitted videotaped telefluoroscopy examinations between the hospitals. He proposed a network that would connect hospitals and physicians' offices so that radiologic information could be exchanged more quickly to referring physicians. The early teleradiology and "telehealth" projects were funded by the U.S. government with the hope that interactive telecommunications would improve access to medical services for those isolated in rural areas. The results of these early programs were encouraging, but many of the projects were discontinued when the funding ran out. It is important to note that the early teleradiology systems were underutilized by the primary care physicians. Today this is still a difficult problem to overcome in practical applications of teleradiology.

In 1970 Murphy and associates reported their results in transmitting images of chest films from patients with tuberculosis via a microwave link.[1,3] The three chest physicians who viewed the radiographs were instructed to assume that any abnormality was produced by tuberculosis. Their results were compared with those of the radiologist who viewed the transmitted images. There was agreement in

77 percent of the cases; the discrepancy is comparable with interobserver variations among radiologists viewing film images directly.[4,5]

In 1972 another study showed that slow scan television techniques could be used to transmit static nuclear radiology images for interpretation,[1,6] although this system was judged inadequate for conventional radiology studies. In this study transmitted positive results were interpreted correctly, but there was a tendency to interpret negative results as equivocal or positive. Still, the study encouraged the use of teleradiology techniques to expand the availability of nuclear radiology.

In 1975 the results were reported of a study on a 4-MHz bandwidth, 525-line television system for radiologic use,[1,7] in which 100 radiographs were evaluated by five experienced radiologists. These evaluators provided interpretations that were said to be of "acceptable accuracy."[1] The report concluded that with further improvements in the system, removal of the residual difference between teleradiology and classic direct film viewing could be expected.

In 1981 Roberts reported a study that compared directly viewed conventional radiographs of the chest with slow scan television images transmitted by phone line[1,8] with respect to visualization of the minor fissure. The minor fissure was seen in 30 percent of the transmitted images and in 97 percent of the directly viewed radiographs, which led to the conclusion that current slow scan television systems were not adequate for use in radiologic consultations. This study obviously was focusing on an anatomic feature that requires very high spatial resolution. The resolution of current teleradiologic systems is discussed more extensively below.

Another teleradiology study was conducted in northern Quebec in 1981.[1,9] Conventional radiologic studies were transmitted via a Canadian satellite, ANIK-B. The system had a resolution of 340 horizontal lines and a true bandwidth of 3 Mhz. Four participating radiologists gave the correct interpretations from

television images in 81 percent of the first 39 selected cases; this increased to 93 percent after they had had 3 months of experience using the system. On the whole, the radiologists were satisfied with the television system.

TECHNICAL DESCRIPTION OF A DIGITAL TELERADIOLOGY SYSTEM

A large number of telecommunications techniques are available using laser fiberoptic systems, microwave links, or satellite relay networks. The problem with these techniques is the high cost of using them to transmit radiologic images, but their advantage is the high speed with which images can be transmitted. Currently the most economical transmission mode is the standard phone line.

The typical phone-based digital teleradiology (DTR) system uses a standard film illuminator mounted horizontally. A conventional screen-film system that has medium to wide contrast latitude is preferred for the transmission of conventional radiologic examinations such as chest, abdomen, and extremities. Most films used in the hard copy formatting of nuclear radiology, ultrasound, computed tomography (CT), and magnetic resonance imaging (MRI) work well on low cost DTR systems. The film to be transmitted is placed on the illuminator, and this image is focused onto the active element of a video camera mounted above the view box. An optical zoom lens, typically an 11- to 110-mm lens with a minimum f-stop value of 1.8, is mounted on the front of the video camera. The DTR system usually has a setup mode where the film can be viewed directly on the video screen while the f-stop and zoom of the optical lens are adjusted. The video camera uses charge-coupled device (CCD) technology and is linked to a microcomputer by a shielded cable.

The analog image from the video camera is digitized using an analog-to-digital (A/D) converter with 512×512 pixel elements 8 bits deep for a gray scale of 256 levels. A total of 2,097,152 bits of information per image must be stored in the microcomputer memory. The digital image can then be displayed on a video display screen, and another film can be put on the illuminator for the next digitization process. The digital images are stored in the computer memory or on a disc drive if necessary. The number of images that can be saved is limited by the size of the computer memory and the capacity of the disc drive. If necessary, additional images can be stored on a new diskette.

Usually some basic image processing features are available in a DTR system that can be used to process a digital image shown on the display CRT screen. These include the ability to adjust the gray scales, window level and window width, and reverse gray scale and to zoom onto an area of interest. It is important to realize that the best way to see greater detail in the image is to optically zoom onto the area of

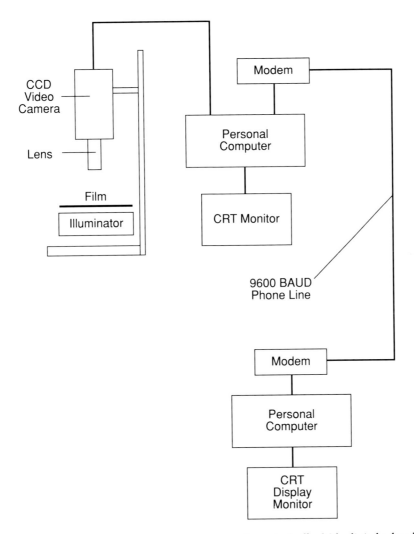

Fig. 4-1. Relationships between the major components of a typical affordable digital teleradiology system.

interest on the original radiograph before the image is digitized rather than to have the computer magnify an area in an image that only has 512×512 pixel resolution. Additional image processing features, such as edge enhancement, and special contrast manipulations, such as Γ correction and histogram equalization, are available on some DTR systems.

The stored image is transmitted over a conventional phone line via a high speed modem. The typical maximum phone line transmission rate is 9600 baud. The image is received by another microcomputer at the other end of the phone line and is displayed on the video display terminal of the receiving microcomputer, which is usually located in the radiologist's home or office. Figure 4-1 shows the typical components of a phone-based DTR system.

RECENT EXPERIENCE WITH DIGITAL TELERADIOLOGY SYSTEMS

There are both advantages and disadvantages to a phone-based teleradiology system ($512 \times 512 \times 8$ bit) when used in a busy private practice. In 1983 Curtis and colleagues described the results of a field trial using teleradiology in a federal health care environment,[10] which included 4,028 interpretations of film and video images by 30 military and civilian radiologists over a 6-month period. The data were transferred from four clinics to a medical center by DTR techniques similar to those described earlier. The films were digitized to a $512 \times 512 \times 8$ bit format, and the images were transferred over a standard telephone line at 9600 baud. The film and video readings were reviewed, and in 160 cases (4 percent) the video reading and the film reading were considered to be discrepant, although 82 of these discrepancies were considered insignificant or could be attributed to differences in terminology. In the remaining 78 cases (1.9

percent) there was substantive disagreement between the video and film readings.

This study indicated that the video interpretations had greater sensitivity and less specificity than the film interpretations. The accuracy of the video interpretation findings was 72.6 percent and that of the film findings was 75.1 percent; the accuracy of the impressions for video and film readings was 76.5 and 80.5 percent, respectively. Thus the film readings were more accurate but only by a small margin. The authors point out that the results of this study are affected by the large number of normal patients examined and by the large number of common pathologic abnormalities that existed in this particular population. However, their results were very encouraging for the increased use of low cost teleradiology systems.

In 1987 Kagetsu et al. reported their experience with a teleradiology system to cover more than one emergency room using a single on-call radiologist.[11] Attending radiologists reviewed 919 video and film examinations. The video images were in a $512 \times 512 \times 8$ bit format and were transferred over a standard phone line at 9600 baud, and a data compression ratio of $2.5:1$ was used for the transmitted data. The measured spatial resolution of the transmitted images was 0.6 lp/mm for the 14×17 inch film and 4 lp/mm for a 5.1×7.3 cm area. The transmission time averaged 2 minutes 50 seconds for a conventional chest radiograph. The transmitted images included 909 plain film radiographs and 10 CT scans.

Of the plain radiologic examinations, 22 had no follow-up, and of the remaining 897 cases, clinically significant discrepancies were found in 5.9 percent (53 cases). An inadequate DTR image caused 1.6 percent of the discrepant examinations, and reader error or interobserver variability caused 4.3 percent. There were more DTR reader errors than film reader errors; this is in part attributable to less experience in using the DTR system by the DTR readers.

The problems identified in the inadequate DTR images were overpenetrated films, limited contrast resolution, and limited spatial resolution. Among the ways suggested by the authors to avoid inadequate DTR images are: (1) to repeat overpenetrated films rather than transmitting them and (2) to use wide latitude film and a brighter transilluminator for film transmission. Transilluminator light has been limited because of the danger of damaging the video camera. The transmission of a gray scale with the DTR images similar to that on many CT images would help the radiologists to make proper adjustments to home monitors.

Certain applications, such as visualization of the pleural line in a large pneumothorax or detection of small abdominal calcifications, pose difficult problems with DTR images at the current spatial resolution of 512×512 pixels. Improved resolution in the apices of the thorax can be obtained by optically zooming the image with a zoom lens prior to transmitting the image; however, the transmission time for a zoomed image of each apex and the posteroanterior and lateral examination would increase the total transmission time to 14 minutes and 50 seconds per chest examination on the system used by Kagetsu et al. It cannot be overemphasized that the original films must be reviewed as soon as practical when using DTR systems. Microwave and fiberoptic image transmission techniques can greatly reduce transmission times for conventional radiography and CT examinations, but these techniques are expensive and do not solve the resolution problem.

My experience in using modest resolution DTR systems to provide emergency room radiology coverage between midnight and 7:00 A.M. is similar to that described by Kagetsu et al.[11] The number of reader errors exceed the number of inadequate DTR images. The number of discrepancies between the digital image reading and the original film reading is not great, but every discrepancy may be significant. Because of the unavoidable discrepancy rate in DTR systems, all DTR readings done in our practice are reviewed at 7:00 A.M., with the original film images used to determine if any discrepancies are present, in which case the emergency room and/or referring physician are contacted immediately. It is important that both the radiologist and the referring physician be aware of the limitations of teleradiology coverage if this technique is to be effective in clinical use.

The pneumothorax provides a good example, as this condition can easily be missed by a non-zoomed DTR image. The referring physician can often direct the radiology technician to transmit a zoomed area of the film, such as the apex of the lung. In my practice the advantages of the DTR system are great, as it enables one radiologist to cover three hospital emergency rooms simultaneously. The radiologist on call may spend all night working at the one hospital with a busy trauma center and still provide imaging expertise to the less busy emergency rooms of the other two hospitals. As the volume of examinations increases to the point that the low-cost teleradiology system cannot transmit the images fast enough to the covering radiologist, it becomes economically viable to place a second radiologist on call. The DTR enables a busy radiology practice to provide 24 hour per day coverage to many hospitals and clinics whose volume does not justify full-time in-house radiologists for around-the-clock coverage. As has been pointed out by Page et al. and Kagetsu et al., it is important to have the radiology technologists thoroughly trained at each site, the referring physicians aware that a teleradiology system is in use, and everyone aware of the limitations of such a system.[9,11] A wide latitude screen-film system works best with current DTR systems, and any underpenetrated or overpenetrated film must be repeated before being transmitted.

ULTRA-HIGH-SPEED TELERADIOLOGY SYSTEM USING NORMAL PHONE LINES

In 1989 Lear and colleagues described the potential for using the new integrated services digital network (ISDN) for transmitting teleradiology images at data rates in excess of

56,000 bits/sec.[12] A modification of their system would be able to transmit at data rates up to 128,000 bits/sec.

The film was placed on an illuminator similar to that in any teleradiology system. A CCD image digitizer was developed to permit digitization at very high spatial and densitometric resolution. A high precision lens was used to focus the radiographic image onto the plane of the CCD array, image lines were scanned mechanically rather than electronically to obtain a scanning resolution up to 2400 × 1800 pixels using 256 gray levels, and a high speed image processing system was developed by using an 80386-based microcomputer. A 1024 × 780 color display was used. This computer was interfaced with the ISDN phone line, and the system was used to transmit images to a remote site 15 miles from the medical center. The system enabled 512 × 512 images to be digitized in 2 seconds, 1024 × 1024 images in 6 seconds, and 1800 × 2400 in 20 seconds. The signal-to-noise ratio of these images exceeded 55:1.

The microcomputer enabled the user to perform basic image processing functions such as contrast enhancement, image filtering, and image compression. Smoothing, sharpening, or edge detection could be performed on a 1024 × 1024 image in 30 seconds. Panels of four CT, MRI, ultrasound, or nuclear medicine images digitized to 512 × 512 pixels were compressed by a 2:1 ratio and subsequent image transmission time was 15 seconds. Conventional radiographs using 1024 × 1024 pixels were also compressed by a 2:1 ratio and required less than 2 minutes to transmit. This system offers a fivefold increase in speed as compared with previous systems that use phone lines. This means that one can transmit more studies in shorter times and overcome some of the disadvantages of existing teleradiology systems such as long transmission times and reduced spatial resolution. This system can be expanded to transmit data at 128,000 bits/sec, which is approximately 25 to 30 percent the speed of expensive satellite data transmission systems.

SUMMARY

Affordable telephone-based digital teleradiology systems enable a single radiologist to provide coverage to many distant facilities at one time. The cost of these systems is modest as compared with the salaries of additional radiologists. The DTR images have a discrepancy rate of approximately 5 percent, many of the errors actually being reader errors. It is important for anyone using a narrow band system to insist on properly exposed radiographs and to promptly review the original images as soon as practical after transmission. The new ISDN technology may provide an affordable advance in DTR by decreasing the time to transmit high resolution images and providing increased spatial resolution as compared with existing affordable phone-based DTR systems.

REFERENCES

1. Carey LS: Teleradiology: Part of a comprehensive telehealth system. Radiol Clin North Am 23:357, 1985
2. Jutra A: Teleroentgen diagnosis by means of videotape recording (editorial). AJR 82:1099, 1959
3. Murphy RLH, Barber D, Broadhurst A, et al: Microwave transmission of chest roentgenograms. Am Rev Respir Dis 102:771, 1970
4. Yevushalmy J: Relativity of chest radiography diagnosis of pulmonary lesions. Am J Surg 89:231, 1955
5. Godard HL: Studies on the accuracy of diagnostic procedures. AJR 82:25, 1959
6. Webber MM, Corbust HR: Image communication by telephone. J Nucl Med 13:379, 1972
7. Andrus WS, Dreyfuss JR, Jaffer F, et al: Interpretation of roentgenograms via interactive television. Radiology 116:25, 1975
8. Roberts JM, House AM, Canning EM: Comparison of slow scan television and direct viewing of radiographs. Can Assoc Radiol J 32:114, 1981
9. Page G, Gregoire A, Galand C, et al: Teleradiology in northern Quebec. Radiology 140:361, 1981

10. Curtis DJ, Gayler BW, Gitlin JN, Harrington MB: Teleradiology: Results of a field trial. Radiology 149:415, 1983

11. Kagetsu NJ, Zulauf DRP, Ablow RC: Clinical trial of digital teleradiology in the practice of emergency room radiology. Radiology 165:551, 1987

12. Lear JL, Manco-Johnson M, Feyerabend A, et al: Ultra-high speed teleradiology with ISDN technology. Radiology 171:862, 1989

TECHNICAL ASPECTS

5

An Overview of Digital Radiography

Stephen Balter

INTRODUCTION

Digital radiography (DR) is the application of digital image handling and processing techniques to projection radiography. The image produced by any radiographic system may be characterized in terms of its spatial resolution, contrast scale, and noise properties. In projection radiography, spatial resolution is a convolution of the properties of the x-ray focal spot, the effects of patient motion, and the intrinsic resolution of the detector. The contrast scale of the image is a convolution of the subject contrast produced by the interaction of the beam with the patient and detector as well as by the gray scale mapping characteristics of the detector and display. Noise arises from the quantum nature of the beam as well as from structural and statistical effects in system components such as the detector.

Various detectors are used to capture the modulated x-ray beam and transform it into an analog or digital image. The separation of image acquisition, image processing, and image display permits optimization of each component of the imaging chain. This separation is one of the major advantages of digital imaging systems. This chapter discusses some of the special considerations related to digital projection radiography as well as some of the more general considerations associated with the processing and display of any digital radiologic image.

IMAGE ACQUISITION

A projection radiograph is formed by using one of the three principal geometries shown in Figure 5-1, namely, projection of a cone of radiation onto a two-dimensional detector, projection of a fan of radiation onto a one-dimensional detector, and projection of a pencil of radiation onto a point detector. Many other

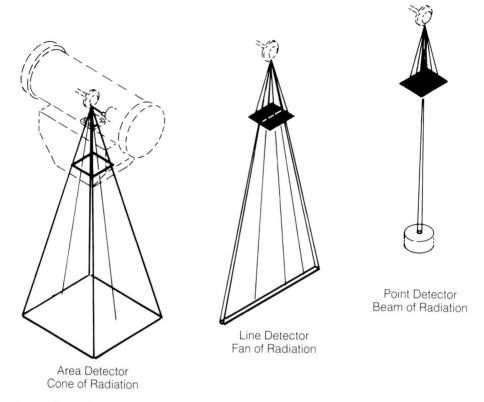

Fig. 5-1. Radiographic projection geometries — cone, fan, and line. As the solid angle decreases, scatter decreases and acquisition time increases.

imaging variants exist. For example, a scanning slit can be used to project an image onto an areal detector (i.e., a sheet of film) line by line. For the fan and pencil beam modes of image formation, appropriate means are used to move the beam-detector assembly relative to the patient.

At the end of each of these image acquisition processes, a two-dimensional transmission image of a patient or other object has been formed and detected. The useful information is carried by spatial and temporal modulations of the detected signal. In the case of any kind of scanned system, a second temporal modulation of the signal may be superimposed on the primary modulations by the scanning motion and may cause clinically significant distortions of the image. As the solid angle of the instantaneous x-ray beam is decreased, the effects of scatter are reduced, which potentially increases the signal-to-noise ratio (SNR) in the modulated x-ray beam. However, the effective efficiency of the x-ray tube decreases as the beam's solid angle is decreased, which results in increased thermal loading on the tube, requiring a larger focal spot and usually prolongs the exposure time. These factors may result in increased geometric or motion unsharpness.

Presently, no narrow pencil beam systems are used for clinical projection radiography. A fat pencil, or a narrow cone, is used in the scanned equalized system developed by Plewes[1] and Wandtke.[2] A novel multiple beam scanning equalization radiography (AMBER) system, was described in 1988 by Vlasbloem and Schultze Kool.[3] These systems modulate the intensity of the x-ray beam spatially ahead of the patient so as to reduce the latitude (dynamic range) of the beam delivered to the detector.

Linear arrays of detectors, used with a fan of radiation, have evolved from the fan beam geometries used with third and fourth generation computed tomography (CT) systems. An example of such a system is the digital chest unit developed by Tesic et al.,[4,5] the geometry of which is shown in Figure 5-2. Each detector in this class of system usually has its own signal amplifier and conditioner. Individual or multiplexed analog-to-digital (A/D) converters are assigned to each channel. By placing energy-sensitive detectors in series, it is possible to construct a system that produces energy-dependent images in near real time.[6] Fan beam systems (either single or dual detector) have potential imaging problems, including a relatively low spatial resolution because of the large number of separate detectors required and a kymographic distortion of the image resulting from anatomic motion during the scanning interval. A profound advantage of fan beam systems is that in practice they are the only ones that routinely use slot geometry for radiographic scatter suppression. This results in superior scatter rejection and improved signal-to-noise ratio.

Important parameters of the modulated x-ray beam include its absolute intensity and intensity range, its SNR, and its spatial resolution. An ideal detector will transform all the information content of the modulated beam into either the analog or digital domain.[7,8] Suboptimum conversion anywhere in the system can cause an increase in noise, which results in an irreversible decrease of SNR with a consequent loss of accessible information content. Image processing cannot improve the image quality or information content beyond that in the detected x-ray beam or compensate for these irreversible losses. Image processing may, however, influence the perceptibility of clinically relevant structures.[9-15]

Figure 5-3 illustrates the effects of improper ranging in the analog domain. If potentially useful information is captured in either the horizontal region of the detector's characteristic curve, it is irretrievably lost because of the impossibility of restoring contrast in regions where the stored image has essentially zero contrast. A similar data loss can occur in a digital system, as illustrated in Figure 5-4. The rounded toe and shoulder of analog transfer functions ordinarily give regions of limited image capture, which are usually not present in digital systems. In particular, the shoulder region of film curves is accessible to (and used by) radiologists by means of bright lights. The abrupt white clipping of digital images looks enough like the natural clipping due to film fog to give the observer some basis of relating digital images to the more conventional film images. Black clipping, on the other hand, causes objects to "disappear" in a way that is outside of normal radiographic experience. This effect can be very confusing and occasionally disorienting.

There are engineering and practical elements that cause the analog or digital image to retain less total information than that present in the modulated x-ray beam. Some of these elements are related to the intrinsic nature of the specific image conversion technology. In

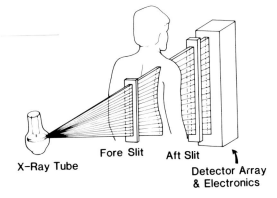

Fig. 5-2. Experimental digital chest radiographic device. Note the use of fan beam geometry. (Courtesy of Picker Medical Systems, Highland Heights, OH.)

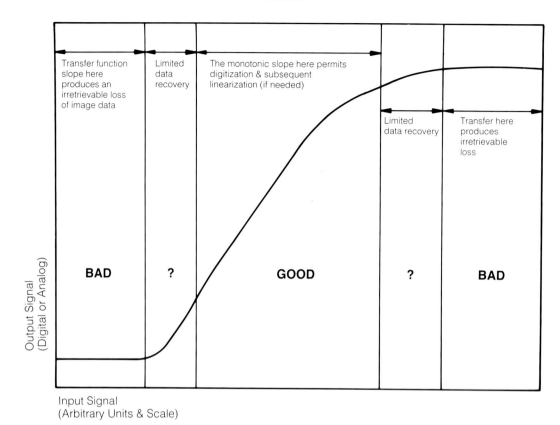

Fig. 5-3. Gray scale transfer function for an analog imaging system. Note the characteristic rounded toe and shoulder.

the digital domain the limit on retained information results from the desire to minimize the number of bits needed to represent an image. The loss of "information" in an absolute sense may or may not affect the clinical information content of a particular image — each situation must be evaluated on its own merits. Thus it is to be expected that digital imaging systems optimized for different purposes will handle images of widely varying matrix sizes and bit depths.

If a full-size chest radiograph is represented by 50-μ pixels, corresponding to a limiting resolution of 10 line pairs per millimeter (lp/mm), 60 megapixels would be required to cover the image area. A simple logarithmic digitization of the x-ray intensity, with allowances for the real dynamic range of the chest and with additional guard bits to give some

measure of exposure latitude, brings the total to around 1000 megabits per image. Given the present realities of storage costs and system bandwidths, such representations are too large for practical purposes. Compromises are sought in the size of the acceptable matrix size[16] and pixel bit depth. The matrix size should be selected on the basis of the required system resolution and the required field of view. Acceptable matrices range from 128 × 128 to 4096 × 4096, with 512 × 512 to 2048 × 2048 being most common. Smaller matrices will yield the same spatial resolution for smaller fields of view. The bit depth of the image should be selected on the basis of an acceptable signal-to-noise ratio. If the quantization level is too coarse relative to the structure and noise content of the final image, then pseudocontouring will result; if it is too fine,

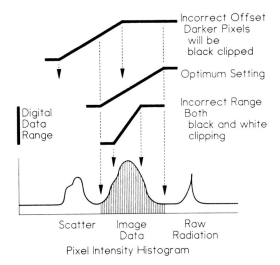

Fig. 5-4. The intensity histogram of an analog image. Improper A/D conversion can result in considerable irretrievable data loss.

then bits are wasted on recording noise. Clinical images require between 8 and 14 bits for image data.

Image intensifier video chains are the radiation transducers used in most digital fluorographic (DF) systems, the most common of which are those specialized for the performance of digital subtraction angiography (DSA).[17] The block diagram of a generic DF system is shown in Figure 5-5. A single-mode or multimode image intensifier is used to convert a radiographic image into optical format, the video chain converts the image into a serial analog electrical signal, and finally an A/D converter produces the digital image. Such a system has numerous electronic processing circuits that affect image quality, some by directly influencing the radiographic operating conditions (e.g., automatic brightness control and automatic exposure termination) and others by manipulating the optical and electrical characteristics of the image (e.g., servo control of the system's optical apertures and automatic gain control in the video chain). More complex feedback control loops provide direct coupling between the video and radiographic systems. The purpose of this design is to transform all the useful information into the working range of the A/D converter. Control of the intensity of the light entering the system's cameras permits the operator to select a working dose level that provides an appropriate level of quantum mottle.

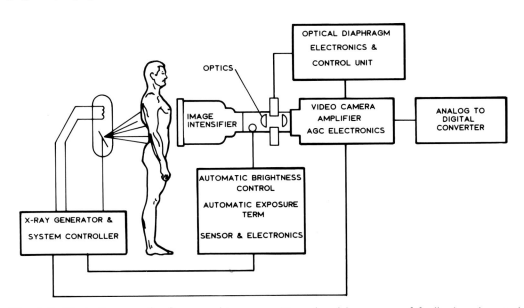

Fig. 5-5. Block diagram of a fluorographic system. Note the elaborate use of feedback and control elements.

The use of multimode image intensifiers is an example of the principle of zooming the image so that the clinically important field of view fills the entire useful aperture. Radiographic magnification produces a similar effect by increasing the apparent size of the object until it fills the entire physical aperture. Zooming of the image intensifier yields improvements in spatial resolution (including "smaller" pixel sizes) as the field of view is reduced (Fig. 5-6). Many clinical fluoroscopic and fluorographic applications do not simultaneously require fine spatial resolution and a large field of view. In these cases the appropriate use of image intensifier zoom and corresponding radiation beam restriction to the smallest relevant field of view maximizes available spatial resolution of any given image matrix while minimizing scatter degradation of the SNR. Even though the input dose in the center of the field increases with decreasing field size because of less geometric minification within the image intensifier, if the optics are correctly set, the patient's integral dose is independent of zoom mode.

The usual system specification of an image intensifier-based digital radiography system includes a 1,000 : 1 SNR, which implies that a 10-bit pixel depth is required to capture and record all the available information in the modulated x-ray beam. The required bit depth may be less when scatter and quantum noise factors are taken into consideration. It is to be noted that the SNR is usually defined in regions of maximum x-ray intensity, and its average value will therefore be a function of the image's intensity histogram. Lightly exposed regions of the image will be noisier than average owing to increased quantum noise and possibly to increased system noise.

The most common radiographic image capture modality is the conventional screen-film system. This system performs all the imaging duties required by most departments, namely, image capture, display, archiving, and communications. In their ninety-fifth year of life film-based systems have evolved to do all these tasks reasonably well. Specialized screen-film systems can achieve a great deal of task-specific image optimization in specific environments; general-purpose systems require more compromises. The principal decision is selection of a system that will give enough contrast for reliable interpretation while preserving enough latitude to encompass both the dynamic range of the body part being imaged as well as providing a margin for exposure errors. As previously shown, portions of a film that are over- or underexposed will lead to irretrievable information loss. The useful dynamic range can be extended by reducing the contrast of the film, which makes the image more difficult to search and interpret visually. If a screen-film system is to be used only as the input to a film digitizer, as has been proposed for the input of radiographs into picture archiving and communications systems (PACS), then a very low contrast transfer characteristic is appropriate to this task because the contrast of the displayed image can be adjusted at a later stage.

Most clinical departments restrict the number of available screen-film speed combinations so that technologist confusion and resulting exposure errors are minimized. The departmental standard screen-film system must possess those resolution, contrast, and noise properties needed for the most demanding examination. The resulting image is likely to have more resolution and to require more than the minimum necessary dose for most examinations. The gray scale transfer function (H and D curve) will be that compromise needed for viewing all examinations reasonably well.

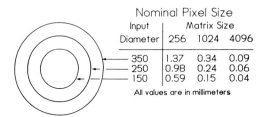

Nominal Pixel Size			
Input	Matrix Size		
Diameter	256	1024	4096
350	1.37	0.34	0.09
250	0.98	0.24	0.06
150	0.59	0.15	0.04

All values are in millimeters

Fig. 5-6. Multimode image intensifier field sizes and corresponding digital fluorographic pixel sizes.

Several alternative aerial detectors have been used for radiography. For example, energy storage detectors consist of sheets of material having the property that when they are irradiated, a portion of the signal is stored as a two-dimensional electron distribution. The system of computed radiography (CR) based upon photostimulable phosphor imaging plate technology developed by the Fuji Photo Film Company[18] is an excellent example of a radiographic imaging system in which an aerial energy storage detector is used to separate primary image capture from other aspects of imaging such as image processing and displaying, thereby permitting separate optimization of image capture and image display parameters.[19-22] The benefits of such a separation of function are available for photofluorographic systems as well as for all other systems in which the image exists in either electronic or digital form.[23,24]

The functional cycle of the photostimulable

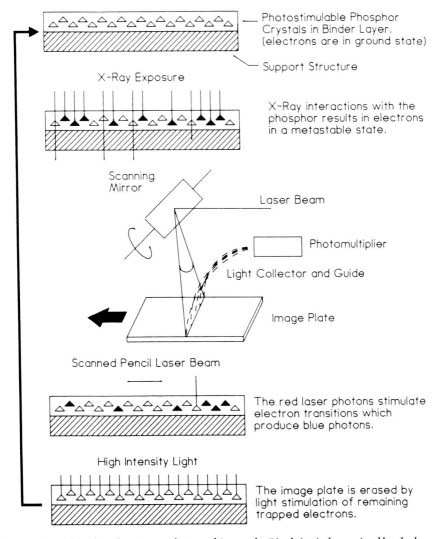

Fig. 5-7. CR stimulable phosphor image plate working cycle. Pixel size is determined by the laser spot size and sampling rate.

energy storage detector is shown in Figure 5-7. Europium dopants create trapping centers in the phosphor, which will trap about half of the signal carrier electrons released in the crystal during irradiation. These traps are relatively stable, and there is little loss of the stored image over several hours. Subsequent irradiation of the phosphor with red light releases a portion of this stored energy as blue fluorescence. The image plate is read out by scanning it with a pencil helium-neon laser beam, and the resulting fluorescence is collected and digitized. An example of the resulting image is shown in Figure 5-8. The raw digital image obtained in this manner may then be processed to produce alternative representations of the data; a sample image pair of a difficult radiographic projection is shown in Figure 5-9. The remaining images in this chapter were all obtained and processed with either the FCR101/PH or PCR/SP computed radiography system.

The dose-response characteristics of the photostimulable phosphor are linear over a dose range of more than four orders of magnitude. With proper setting of the CR system, subject contrast is captured with the same efficiency at "low," "correct," and "high" doses. Figures 5-10 to 5-12 illustrate this point with a skull phantom, for which images were obtained at detector exposures of 1.5×10^{-8}, 7.7×10^{-8}, and 7.7×10^{-7} C/kg (60, 300, and 3000 μR; the 7.7×10^{-8} C/kg (300 μR) exposure corresponds to that required by a 300 to 400 speed screen-film system. The overall contrast and density of the resulting digital radiograph are preserved over this range. The noise characteristics of the low dose image may make it unacceptable for many purposes, but the subject contrast has been captured. At high doses system noise and structure mottle dominate x-ray quantum noise. Once this occurs, further increases in dose will not lead to direct improvements in

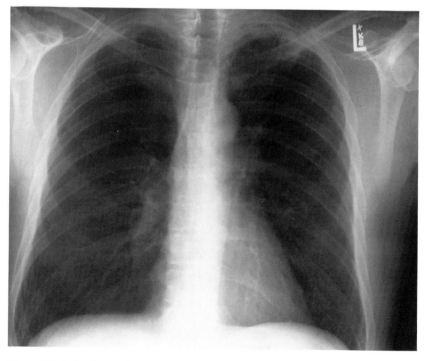

Fig. 5-8. Neutral digital radiograph. Nominal 2100 × 1800 pixels, corresponding to 2.5 lp/mm. Linear gray scale transfer. No unsharp masking.

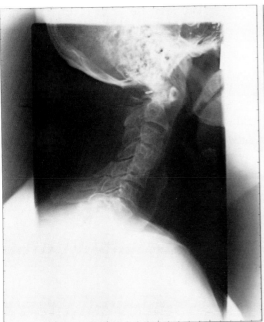 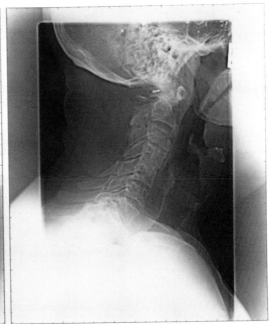

Fig. 5-9. Typical digital image pair produced by the CR system. Different image processing operators were used on each side.

image quality. The stability of contrast and density in the high dose range does, however, yield a clinically important improvement in image uniformity.

There is a subtle but critical implication in this new found freedom in projection radiography. Unacceptably low dose radiographs obtained with conventional screen-film systems are automatically rejected since the films are visibly underexposed. Corresponding CR images may lead to a failure of detection of low contrast targets, which is attributable to the increased noise content of the image. Existing CR systems report a sensitivity number, which is inversely related to the dose received by the imaging plate (IP), on each image. Clinicians and quality assurance officers should be aware of the minimum doses required for specific tasks and be prepared to reject those images whose doses are too low, even though the images may appear to be acceptable. Similarly, doses that are systematically too high should be investigated. Because dose is now a free and important variable, dosimetry information needs to be carried among the image descriptors in the PACS environment.

IMAGE HANDLING

Image handling and image processing are two distinct concepts, which should be regarded as separate entities. An *image handling* system physically moves or archives images without transforming their properties. An *image processor* takes an input image and produces a transformed output image. Most complete imaging systems have both handling and processing components. For example, when an image is acquired, it undergoes both analog and digital processing (some of which is unintentional) as it is moved from the detector, through the system, in and out of archives, and finally to an analog display device. A few specific considerations related to the design of a

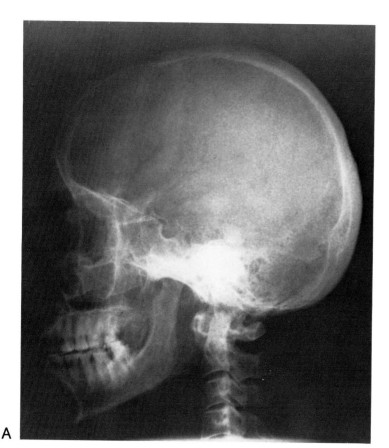

Fig. 5-10. (A) Digital radiograph of a phantom image plate exposure of 3,000 μR. System and structure noise visible. **(B)** A photographic enlargement of the sellar region.

A

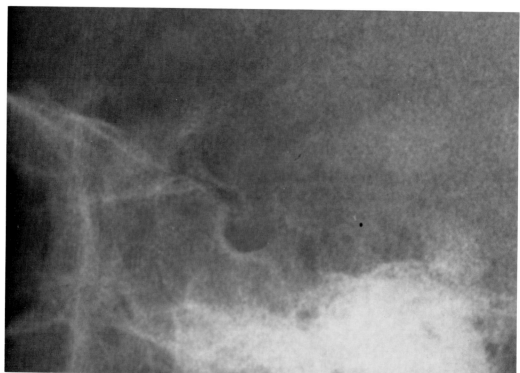

B

Fig. 5-11. (A) Image plate exposure 300 μR. The same image plate was used as in Fig. 5-10. Normal clinical dose range. **(B)** A photographic enlargement of the sellar region.

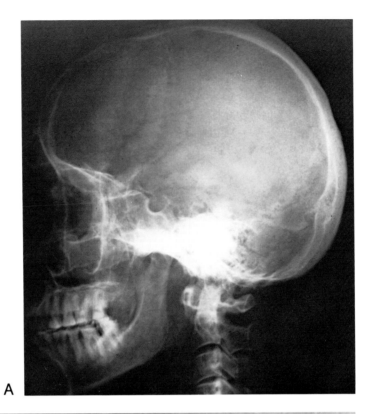

A

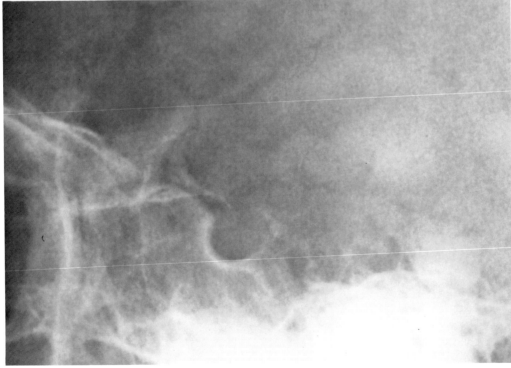

B

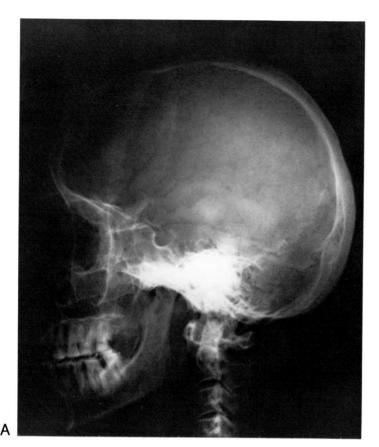

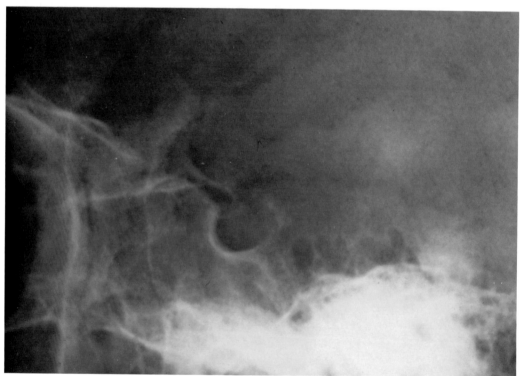

Fig. 5-12. (A) Image plate exposure 60 μR which is below the normal clinical working range. X-ray noise dominates this image. (B) A photographic enlargement of the sellar region.

digital radiography system and its internal image handling will be discussed below. In the clinic the tens of images associated with a typical patient must be collected, archived, communicated, and displayed. The implementation, technology, and economics of PACS are discussed elsewhere[25-27] and in Chapter 8.

In comparison with most data sets handled by computerized means, the raw information content of individual medical images is very high. A single digital image ranges from 0.25 Mbyte in a simple digital fluorograph to about 10 MByte in a high resolution digital radiograph. This has several implications for system design and leads to the use of data compression in many cases. For example, a DR system needs high internal bus, mass storage, and processor speeds. DF systems of smaller matrix size often have the most critical speed requirements because image capture and processing must occur at rates ranging from less than one image per second (fluorography) to 30 images per second (cinefluorography). Digital fluorographs are often viewed and clinically used immediately after acquisition. Digital radiographs are acquired at rates ranging from a few per second (serial changers) to a few per hour. Digital radiographs seldom need to be viewed in less than a few seconds after capture.

Speed at reasonable cost places constraints on the nature of the image structure and the processing algorithms that can be employed. Image matrix size and pixel bit depth are necessarily reduced so as to move images quickly through a system with fixed bandwidth.[28] The elimination of unimportant bits (data compression) should not proceed beyond the point at which the clinical purposes of the examination are compromised. Because medicine is a conservative art, physicians may doubt the integrity of the compressed image if image quality is reduced without consideration of confidence safety margins. Use of high speed image capture and a subsequent slower processing cycle is acceptable provided that the original data capture does not degrade the image and that the complete cycle is fast enough to meet the clinical needs of the examination.

The question of data compression is almost as important to the design of DR systems as it is to the design of PACS systems. Appropriate image compressors are needed to efficiently store digital radiographic, fluorographic, and cinefluorographic images. The raw data bandwidth needed for cinefluorography can exceed 10 megapixels per second for periods exceeding 10 seconds. Image compression algorithms either are totally reversible or produce some irreversible "loss" of image information. Digital radiographs can be reversibly compressed by a factor of around 2.5 and irreversibly compressed to a much greater degree.[29,30]

At present, many physicians are unwilling to work clinically with any image that has undergone an irreversible compression. This may be due only to an unfortunate semantic consequence associated with the word "irreversible" and not to a real limitation of appropriate data compression. The difference between the original and the compressed-decompressed image can be regarded as an additional noise source in the imaging system; a reversible algorithm is free from compression noise, whereas an irreversible algorithm will add some degree of additional noise to the image. If compression noise makes a small contribution compared with other noise sources in the complete imaging system (including x-ray quantum noise), it is likely to be unnoticeable.

IMAGE PROCESSING

The processing of images in a stable and reproducible manner is a major technical and clinical requirement for digital radiography. Digital tools permit image transformations that cannot be achieved in the analog domain. With appropriate processing algorithms, one can improve the perceptibility of clinically significant structures and possibly improve the accuracy of the diagnostic process. However, image processing carried to an extreme will disorient both radiologists and clinicians. In any radiographic setting, there is a need to build strong bridges between the observer's concept of the patient's anatomy and pathology and the visual representation of the observer's mental construct in the image.[31-35]

One must also consider that radiologists have a finite amount of time for routine interpretation of radiographs. The image processor should use prestored algorithms for the computation of optimum output images in most cases, and the processing of most images should be completed prior to viewing. As an example of the trade-offs between processing equipment and observer time, a single observer reading screening chest radiographs in almost any format will miss about 30 percent of the positive findings, which is in part, attributable to the low prevalence of disease in screening populations. The false negative rate can be reduced to around 10 percent by having two radiologists interpret the films separately.[36] It is to be carefully noted that the present use of radiologic images is not a solitary operation — images are discussed between residents and attending physicians, between radiologists and referring physicians, and in clinical conferences. This methodology, while expensive in physician time, reduces the likelihood of a missed finding and improves the transfer of important information from the images and of diagnostic impressions from the radiologist to the responsible clinician.

For interactive image processing to be economically viable, it must perform as well in extracting information about the patient as would double reading but without doubling reader time. There are special cases, such as trauma and surgical planning, in which unlimited observer time is justified. In these cases interactive image processing and other computerized aids may be of vital importance.[37] For this reason digital radiology facilities should have at least one fully equipped workstation available for such tasks. Experience has shown that simple gray scale remapping should be provided on all viewing terminals. These controls are discussed in more detail below.

Multipixel Transformations

The histogram of pixel count vs. pixel value in a digital radiograph is a complicated structure, which is dependent upon the radiographic imaging conditions as well as upon the patient's anatomy and pathology. Histogram analysis can be used to find the regions of valid clinical data within a much wider preliminary search range and thereby maximize the use of available bit depth in the A/D converter (a representation of such a histogram is shown in Fig. 5-4). Histogram equalization techniques, applied between the input and output, are a way of mapping the digital representation of an image so as to make maximum use of the available output gray scale.[38,39] At the present state of the art, optimum histogram analysis requires some a priori information regarding the anatomy and radiographic conditions. The image resulting from full histogram equalization is presently considered too different from the conventional appearance of a radiograph to be useful in routine practice. Global and constrained histogram equalizations are beginning to be used clinically in the digital processing of radiotherapy port films[40] (JM Balter, personal communication 1988).

Convolution operations can be used to modify the modulation transfer function (MTF) of a digital system. In principle many different convolution filter shapes can be applied to an image, but in practice the need for rapid image throughput currently limits the choice for clinical use to variants of the square kernel unsharp mask algorithm. Other desirable filters will no doubt be implemented as image processor bandwidths increase.

It is worthwhile to look at the unsharp mask operator in some detail. Each pixel in the image becomes the "target" pixel in turn, and an average is taken of all the pixels in a square region of the original image surrounding the target pixel. A weighted sum is then constructed by combining this average with the target pixel value. The size of the averaging region and the weighting factor are usually taken as adjustable factors. As the requirements for image processing speed increase, the size of the averaging region usually decreases owing to image processor bandwidth limitations. Digital fluoroscopic systems usually average over a maximum mask region of only a few pixels while slower digital radiographic systems permit use of a maximum mask region of more than 100 pixels on a side. The selection of the appropriate unsharp mask size and weighting factor is highly task-dependent. Figure 5-13 illustrates the influence of unsharp mask kernel size on the appearance of a chest radiograph. The weighting factor used for these examples is larger than those used clinically.

Noise Reduction

Algorithms exist for minimizing the perceived noise in digital images; most of these algorithms are spatial frequency filters and are effective only when the spatial frequencies of a clinically useful signal and those of noise can be separated. For example, an algorithm that replaces single pixel noise spikes with an average of nearest neighbors is effective because the spike's signal intensity is located in those spatial frequencies corresponding to a region of low modulation transfer function of the total imaging system. To use an audio analogy, noise filters essentially remove the high frequencies from the image and are more effective in cleaning up speech than music because the high frequency content of speech is low relative to that of music or noise.

The visual effect of noise is enhanced by the unsharp mask operator. In practice, the application of unsharp masking is adapted to the potential interference of enhanced noise with viewing conditions. Data such as neonatal chest images are often computed with little or no unsharp masking because enhanced noise from the unsharp mask operator matches the frequency content of certain types of interstitial lung disease. Unsharp masking in these cases would remove diagnostically useful information. In processing chest radiographs to search for nodules, a great deal of visual noise may be accepted in return for the enhanced visualization of nodules. The same algorithm would be inappropriate when the clinical question is one of interstitial disease because the unsharp mask operator increases the visualization of diagnostically irrelevant anatomy.

Single Pixel Operations

The ability to map the digital representation of a pixel to an arbitrary gray scale value is a key tool available in a digital radiography system. It is possible to produce digital images with gray scale characteristics that are chemically and physically impossible to achieve with either film or pure analog computational technologies. A well designed system can produce the same subjective representation (on the output of a fixed parameter hard copy or soft copy display digital system) that is produced by any given radiographic film. However, the capability to track a variable cathode-ray tube image so that its corresponding hard copy is an exact subjective match in the eyes of the radiologist is not within the present state of the art.

Users of digital imaging systems should be aware that gray scale transformations are more subtle than the simple window and level controls found on many display devices. It is possible to transform the data so that the "level shift" occurs along either the horizontal or vertical axis. Only when the transfer function is linear with a slope of unity will these two transformations have the same effect on the image. As shown in Figure 5-14, if a system has a sigmoidal gray scale transfer function, a simple vertical level shift changes the brightness (density) of an image but does not affect the relative contrast of different structures. A horizontal shift (corresponding to a milliampere seconds [mAs] change in radiography) affects both local brightness (density) and local contrast. Adjustment of the brightness and contrast controls on the monitor is highly nonlinear. It is good practice to set these controls to properly calibrated positions and to use digital gray scale transformations to adjust the

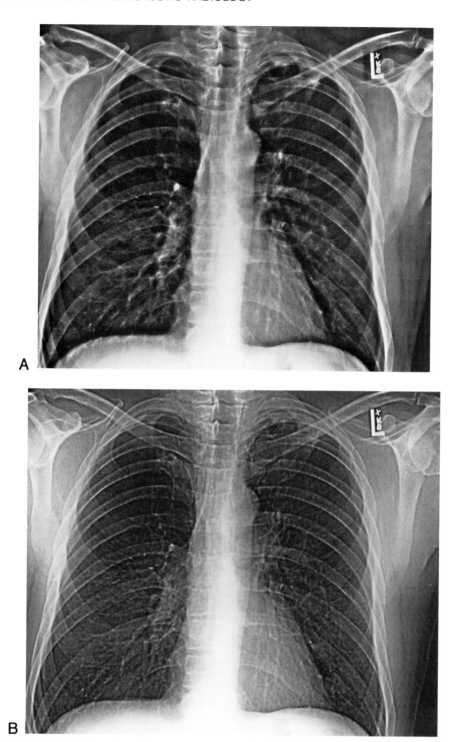

Fig. 5-13. The effect of unsharp masking on a digital chest radiograph. Pixel size: 0.2 mm. The weighting factor is 6 for all four images, which is greater than required for most clinical applications. **(A)** Kernel: 99 × 99 pixels. **(B)** Kernel: 41 × 41 pixels. *(Figure continues.)*

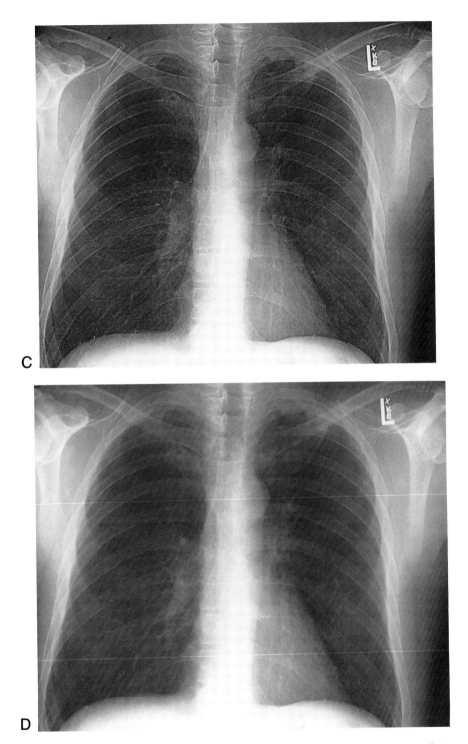

Fig. 5-13 *(Continued).* **(C)** Kernel: 21 × 21 pixels. **(D)** Kernel: 3 × 3 pixels.

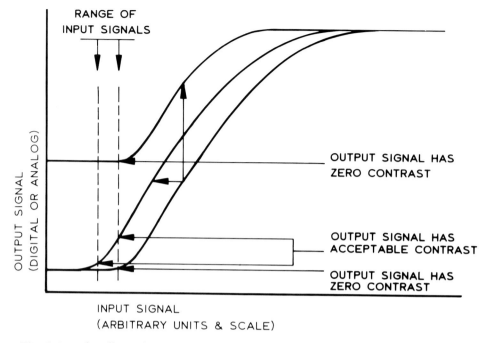

Fig. 5-14. The effects of horizontal and vertical density shifts on local contrast and density.

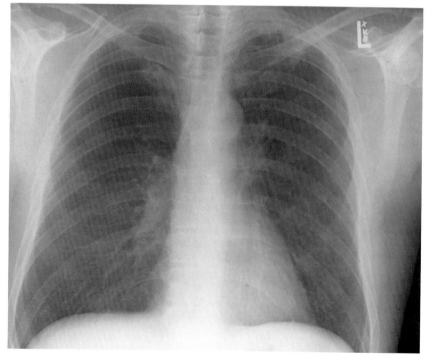

A

Fig. 5-15 (A) Sample radiograph with lowered contrast and density horizontally shifted toward low values. *(Figure continues.)*

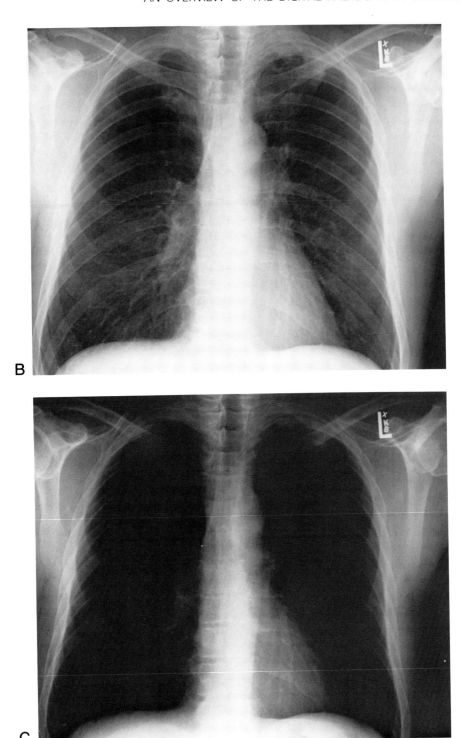

Fig. 5-15 *(Continued).* **(B)** Same radiograph with clinically optimized contrast and density. **(C)** Same radiograph with increased contrast and density horizontally shifted toward high values.

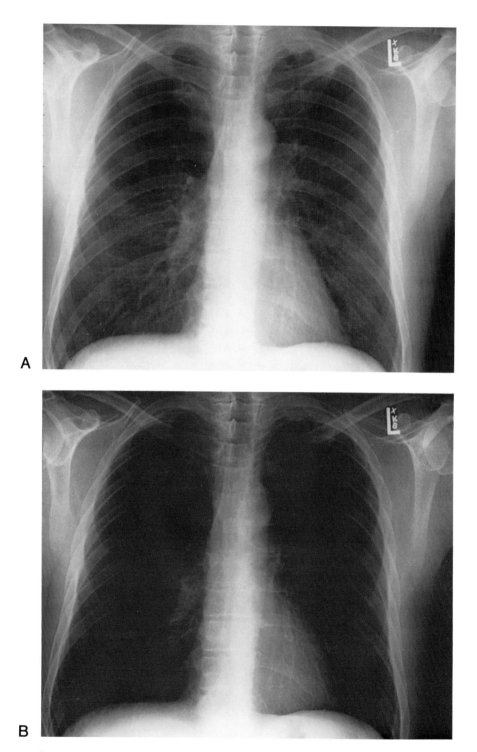

Fig. 5-16. **(A)** CR chest image displayed by using clinically optimized chest imaging parameters. **(B)** CR chest image displayed by using clinically optimized abdominal imaging parameters. *(Figure continues.)*

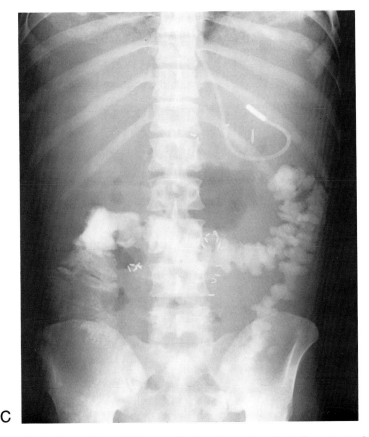

C

Fig. 5-16 *(Continued).* **(C)** CR abdominal image displayed by using clinically optimized chest imaging parameters. *(Figure continues.)*

appearance of the image. Figure 5-15 illustrates the effects of changing global contrast and applying a horizontal density shift on the appearance of the same image. Here again, the images use exaggerated transformation parameters for demonstration purposes.

Figure 5-16 presents examples of empirically optimized displays for chest and abdominal radiography. The profound effects of using incorrect display functions are also shown in this series. It should be obvious that digital display functions need to be selected with at least as much care as is used in selection of a film type for conventional radiography. The users of task-specific image displays should not

be surprised that an incorrect selection leads to suboptimum image quality.

Difference Imaging

Because of the stability of digital image processors, the first routine application of digital radiography was the subtraction of fluorographic angiographic images. A mask image was obtained prior to contrast injection and was later subtracted from the contrast image. Subtraction imaging emphasizes the difference between a given image and a reference image. These subtraction images are intended to demonstrate temporal or energy differences be-

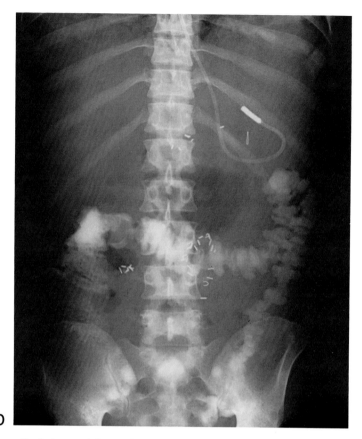

Fig. 5-16 *(Continued).* **(D)** CR abdominal image displayed by using clinically optimized abdominal imaging parameters.

tween the two original images. Since all changes between the two images are shown, radiographic exposure conditions as well as image processing parameters must be controlled so as to minimize unwanted contributions to the difference image.

The difference image has unusual properties in relation to either of the two original images, including a reduction in global signal intensity and an increase in both global and regional noise intensity. The subtraction process removes common mode information, and therefore there is less total signal in the difference image than in either original. Stochastic noise, because it is not in common mode in the two images, is quadratically summed by the subtraction process. In a situation in which the original images are quantum noise-limited, a ghost, or "noise print," of the subtracted structures is seen in the resultant image.[41]

Subtraction images are of value only when the conspicuity of clinically needed information is improved relative to the original image and to the amplified noise in the subtraction. The formal global SNR of a subtraction is always less than that in either of the two initial images. Since subtraction images represent contrast-amplified small differences between the two original images, they are susceptible to digital contouring artifacts when the digitization steps are too coarse relative to the difference signals.

The stability of DR systems opens the possibility of routine energy difference imaging. In

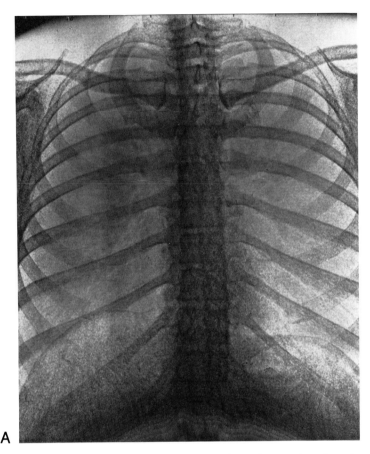

A

Fig. 5-17. Example of an energy subtraction image pair. Additional corrections have been applied for beam hardening, scatter suppression, and noise reduction. **(A)** Soft tissue suppressed. *(Figure continues.)*

such systems, different x-ray spectra are used to acquire each of two images, the differences between which may be exploited to obtain representations in which bone or soft tissue components are suppressed.[42] The presence or absence of calcium in a structure is of considerably diagnostic importance.[43,44] The method for performing such studies using stimulable phosphor image plates was recently described by Ishigaki et al.[45] Figure 5-17 presents examples of an image pair produced by Ergun et al.[46] with either bone or soft tissue suppression. These images were obtained by using a single exposure of two image plates separated by an energy separation filter. The exposure to the image plate cassette was approximately 1.3 × 10^{-7} C/kg (500 μR). Additional corrections have been made to these images for regional beam hardening and for noise and scatter suppression.

CONCLUSION

Digital radiography may be defined by the presence of an image in digital form. It operationally separates different imaging tasks into different system components, therefore making it possible to separately optimize image capture, PACS, the extraction of diagnostic information, and image display. This separation opens up new fields of investigation and

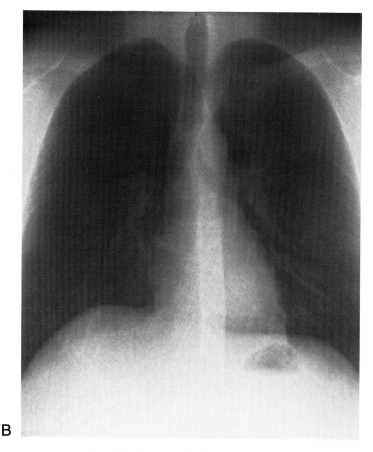

B

Fig. 5-17 *(Continued).* **(B)** Bone suppressed.

development. The end result of such efforts should be the evolution of new digital imaging concepts that maximize diagnostic yield per unit of dose, cost, and physician time.

REFERENCES

1. Plewes DB: A scanning system for chest radiography with regional exposure control: Theoretical considerations. Med Phys 10:654, 1984
2. Wandtke JC: Improved pulmonary nodule detection with scanning equalization radiography. Radiology 169:23, 1988
3. Vlasbloem H, Schultze Kool LJ: AMBER: A scanning multiple beam equalization system for chest radiography. Radiology 169:29, 1988
4. Tesic MM, Sones RA, Morgan DR: Single-slit digital radiography: Some practical considerations. AJR 142:697, 1984
5. Barnes GT, Sones RA, Tesic MM: Digital chest radiography: Performance evaluation of a prototype unit. Radiology 154:801, 1985
6. Fraser RG, Nickey NM, Niklason LT, et al: Calcification in pulmonary nodules: Detection with dual-energy digital radiography. Radiology 160:595, 1986
7. Giger ML, Doi K: Investigation of basic imaging properties in digital radiography. 3. Effect of pixel size on SNR and threshold contrast. Med Phys 12:201, 1985
8. Giger ML, Ohara K, Doi K: Investigation of basic imaging properties in digital radiography. 9. Effect of displayed gray levels on signal detection. Med Phys 13:312, 1986
9. Davis GW, Wallenslager ST: Improvement of

chest region CT images through automated gray-level remapping. IEEE Trans Med Imaging 5:30, 1986

10. Goodman LR, Foley WD, Wilson CR, et al: Pneumothorax and other lung diseases: Effect of altered resolution and edge enhancement on diagnosis with digitized radiographs. Radiology 167:83, 1988

11. Oestmann JW, Kushner DC, Bourgouin PM, et al: Subtle lung cancers: Impact of edge enhancement and gray scale reversal on detection with digitized chest radiographs. Radiology 167:657, 1988

12. Rogowska J, Preston K Jr, Sashin D: Evaluation of digital unsharp masking and local contrast stretching as applied to chest radiographs. IEEE Trans Biomed Eng 35:817, 1988

13. Sakuma H, Takeda K, Hirano T, et al: Plain chest radiograph with computed radiography: Improved sensitivity for the detection of coronary artery calcification. AJR 151:27, 1988

14. Samarasekara MG, Hudson FR: A technique for image density matching in radiotherapy planning radiographs. Br J Radiol 61:697, 1988

15. Sherrier RH, Chiles C, Wilkinson WE, et al: Effects of image processing on nodule detection rates in digitized radiographs: ROC study of observer performance. Radiology 166:447, 1988

16. Fujita H, Giger ML, Doi K: Investigation of basic imaging properties in digital radiography. 12. Effect of matrix configuration on spatial resolution. Med Phys 15:384, 1988

17. Mistretta CA, Crummy AB: Diagnosis of cardiovascular disease by digital subtraction angiography. Science 214:761, 1981

18. Sonoda M, Takano M, Miyahara J, Kato H: Computed radiography using scanning laser stimulated luminescence. Radiology 148:883, 1983

19. Fuhrman CR, Gur D, Good B, et al: Storage phosphor radiographs vs conventional films: Interpreters' perceptions of diagnostic quality. AJR 150:1011, 1988

20. Kangarloo H, Boechat MI, Barbaric Z, et al: Two-year clinical experience with a computed radiographic system. AJR 151:505, 1988

21. Kogutt MS, Jones JP, Perkins DD: Low dose digital computed radiography in pediatric chest imaging. AJR 151:775, 1988

22. Merritt CRB, Matthews CC, Scheinhorn D, Balter S: Digital imaging of the chest. J Thorac Imaging 1:1, 1985

23. Balter S: On the work of the radiologist—separation of image capture from image display. Acta Radiol 29:257, 1988

24. Goodman LR, Wilson CR, Foley WD: Digital radiography of the chest: Promises and problems. AJR 150:1241, 1988

25. Cho PS, Huang HK, Tillisch J, Kangarloo H: Clinical evaluation of a radiologic picture archiving and communication system for a coronary care unit. AJR 15:823, 1988

26. Mezrich RS. The implication of PACS for radiology practice. AJR 151:828, 1988

27. DeSimone DN, Kundel HL, Arenson RL, et al: Effect of a digital imaging network on physician behavior in an intensive care unit. Radiology 169:41, 1988

28. Bramble JM, Huang HK, Murphy MD: Image data compression. Invest Radiol 23:707, 1988

29. Lo SC, Huang KH: Radiological image compression: Full-frame bit-allocation technique. Radiology 155:811, 1985

30. Lo SC, Huang HK: Compression of radiological images with 512, 1,024, and 2,048 matrices. Radiology 161:519, 1986

31. Berbaum KS, El-Khoury GY, Franken EA Jr: Impact of clinical history on fracture detection with radiography. Radiology 168:507, 1988

32. Berbaum KS, Franken EA Jr, Dorfman DD, Barloon TJ: Influence of clinical history upon detection of nodules and other lesions. Invest Radiol 23:48, 1988

33. Cowen AR, Hartley PJ, Workman A: The computer enhancement of digital grey-scale fluorographic images. Br J Radiol 61:492, 1988

34. MacMahon H, Metz CE, Doi K, et al: Digital chest radiography: Effect on diagnostic accuracy of hard copy, conventional video, and reversed gray scale video display formats. Radiology 168:669, 1988

35. Swensson RG: The effects of clinical information on film interpretation: Another perspective. Invest Radiol 23:56, 1988

36. Hessel SJ, Herman PG, Swenson RG: Improving performance by multiple interpretation of chest radiographs: Effectiveness and cost. Radiology 127:589, 1978

37. Getty DJ, Picket RM, D'Orsi CJ, Swets JA:

Enhanced interpretation of diagnostic images. Invest Radiol 23:240, 1988

38. Dhawan AP, Buelloni G, Gordon R: Enhancement of mammographic features by optimal adaptive neighborhood image processing. IEEE Trans Med Imaging 5:8, 1986

39. Braunstein EM, Capek P, Buckwalter K, et al: Adaptive histogram equalization in digital radiography of destructive skeletal lesions. Radiology 166:883, 1988

40. Wilenzick RM, Merritt CRB, Balter S: Megavoltage portal films using computed radiographic imaging with photostimulable phosphors. Med Phys 14:389, 1987

41. Balter S, Ergun D, Tscholl E, et al: Digital subtraction angiography: Fundamental noise characteristics. Radiology 152:195, 1984

42. Alvarez RE, Mascovski A: Energy-selective reconstructions in x-ray computed tomography. Phys Med Biol 21:733, 1976

43. Ishigaki T, Sakuma S, Ikeda M: One-shot dual-energy subtraction chest imaging with computed radiography: Clinical evaluation of film images. Radiology 168:67, 1988

44. Asaga T, Chiyasu S, Mastuura H, et al: Breast imaging: Dual-energy projection radiography with digital radiography. Radiology 164:869, 1987

45. Ishigaki T, Sakuma S, Horikawa Y, et al: One-shot dual-energy subtraction imaging. Radiology 161:271, 1986

46. Ergun D, Mistretta CA, Brown DE: Dual-energy phosphor cassette for computed radiography. Presented at the 74th Annual Meeting of the Radiological Society of North America, Chicago, 1988

6

Digital Radiography Using Storage Phosphors

Ralph Schaetzing
Bruce R. Whiting
Anthony R. Lubinsky
James F. Owen

INTRODUCTION

Although many of the predictions made in the late 1970s about the ubiquity of the "all-digital department" by 1990 have not come true, the use of digital technology in medical imaging has unquestionably increased since that time. The failure to realize these early expectations is as much due to issues of economic viability as it is to the technical complexity of digital imaging systems and to concerns about their diagnostic utility. These issues continue to be the subject of extensive research and development.

The addition of a digital section to the medical image chain (Fig. 6-1) has some important implications for systems design and performance. In particular, the separation of image capture from image display and the potential benefits resulting from the ability (and need)

to manipulate the data require a different strategy for system optimization and the selection of design trade-offs. Furthermore, there are many more variables to consider in the evaluation of diagnostic utility on the basis of observer performance studies.

In the area of projection radiography, which still accounts for the majority of all images generated in radiology departments, a number of digital technologies are challenging the established preeminence of screen-film imaging as an acquisition/display medium. One of these technologies is storage phosphor (SP) imaging. In this chapter we review this promising technology, including its long and interesting history, the fundamentals of system design and operation, and the theoretical and practical characterization of system performance. As far as possible we compare the performance of SP systems with the screen-film

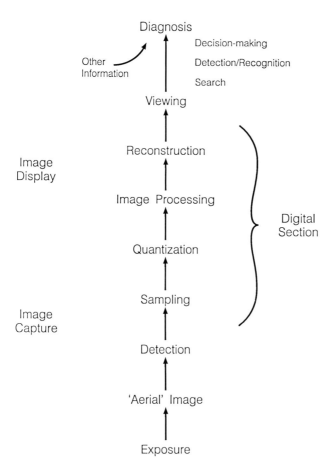

Fig. 6-1. The medical image chain.

systems they are intended to replace. We close with a short discussion of the effects of image processing in digital radiography and some clinical results achieved with SP systems.

Conventional Screen-Film Technology

Perhaps the greatest challenge to the scientists and engineers involved in the development of electronic imaging technologies for projection radiography is to produce a system that can match the image quality, reliability, cost, throughput rate, and relative ease of use of the conventional screen-film/processor/view box system. Today's digital networking, archiving, and soft display technologies, that is, picture archiving and communications sys-

tems (PACS) technology, cannot cost-effectively handle the massive amounts of information contained in projection radiographs. Consequently, the mere fact that an electronic imaging system is digital is not yet sufficient to ensure its success in the medical marketplace for general-purpose radiography.

Film is an exceptionally high quality detector/display combination—it is the "gold standard" with which any electronic projection radiography system will be compared. Furthermore, even though it is a very mature technology, with almost 100 years of development work behind it, significant improvements in screen-film image quality, exposure requirements, and processing speeds are possible and continue to be made. Thus, conventional screen-film radiography provides a "moving target" for the emerging electronic systems.

The procedure for producing a screen-film radiograph is a straightforward one. Radiographic film comes in two basic types, single emulsion and double emulsion. Single-emulsion film has emulsion coated on only one side of a polyester substrate and is used for high resolution applications (e.g., breasts, extremities). Double-emulsion film is coated on both sides of the substrate and is used in applications in which higher speed is desired and somewhat lower resolution can be tolerated (e.g., thorax, abdomen). Inside a radiographic cassette, the emulsion side of a single-sided film is placed in intimate contact with an intensifying ing screen; if double-emulsion film is used, it is sandwiched between two screens. X-rays impinging upon the cassette are absorbed primarily in the intensifying screen(s), which promptly emit light with an intensity proportional to the number of x-rays (and hence the amount of energy) absorbed. Since the film's sensitivity to x-rays is insignificant compared with its sensitivity to light, it is mainly the emission from the intensifying screens that causes the formation of a latent image in the film. The film is subsequently chemically developed, usually in an automated processor, which passes the film through the various chemical baths and washes, and is finally displayed on a view box.

The detailed physics and chemistry of the photographic process cannot be done justice to in this short chapter and have been covered extensively elsewhere.[1] In rather simplified terms, the emulsion consists of small (about 1-μm) crystals of silver halide (primarily silver bromoiodide) embedded in gelatin. Defects on the surface of these grains (Frenkel defects) can provide sites for latent image formation. These defects have a small net positive charge, which can act to trap electrons moving through the crystal. Latent image formation begins when impinging photons free electrons from bromine ions within the crystals and these electrons become trapped at the defect sites. A trapped electron results in a small net negative charge at the site, which can then attract an interstitial silver ion, forming a neutral silver atom and restoring the small net positive charge. This positive charge can again cause another free electron to be trapped, which will attract another interstitial silver ion, and so on. This process results in clumps of silver atoms, or latent image centers, at the site of the crystal defect. During chemical development, all silver ions in the crystals are reduced to form metallic silver, which produces the density in the film. However, this process is much faster in grains containing latent image centers. Thus, if development is halted at the appropriate time, the density in a given area on the film depends upon the number of latent image centers that had been formed in that area, which in turn depends upon the number of photons absorbed.

Because conventional intensifying screens are so similar to the SP screens that will be discussed in this chapter, it is worth saying a few words about their structure and the physical mechanisms that result in the emission of visible or near ultraviolet radiation after x-ray absorption. Radiographic intensifying screens consist of a flexible plastic base coated with a phosphor powder, usually of 1 to 50 μm particle size, embedded in a flexible polymer. Generally, the screens are overcoated with a transparent film that provides protection against abrasion and moisture. Sometimes a reflective layer is placed between the base and the phosphor layer in order to direct emitted light out of the screen. The screens appear white because the large difference in refractive index between the crystals and the polymer gives rise to a significant amount of light scattering within the phosphor layer.

When an x-ray is absorbed in a phosphor particle, some fraction of the energy imparted to the phosphor is emitted in the form of luminescence. Obviously, for a given screen-film combination, the phosphor is chosen and/or the film is designed so that emission will occur at a wavelength to which the film is sensitive.

The larger the fraction of energy that is converted to emitted radiation at the appropriate wavelength, the greater the efficiency of the screen. In general, the more light emitted from a screen for a given x-ray dose, the higher the potential image quality of the screen-film combination. This is true for two reasons. First, a less efficient phosphor requires a faster film for a given x-ray dose, and faster films tend to be more grainy than slower films because of the large silver halide crystals that are required. More importantly, a major fraction of the noise in a medical projection radiograph is *quantum noise* (i.e., noise associated with the statistics of, or variations in, the relatively limited number of x-ray photons per unit area). This noise is compounded by the statistical variation about the mean value of the number of light photons produced per absorbed x-ray. The effect of this variation on image quality becomes (relatively) smaller as the mean value (the *gain*) increases. The importance of keeping this gain large will be discussed again later for SP imaging.

The physical mechanism by which the energy imparted to a phosphor from an absorbed x-ray is transformed into emission is complex.[2] It varies from system to system and in general is not completely understood. For x-ray energies in the diagnostic range, the primary event is the absorption of an incident x-ray photon as the result of a photoelectric interaction between the x-ray and one of the heavier elements in the phosphor. The resulting photoelectron deposits its kinetic energy in the crystal via ionization and excitation. Lower energy characteristic x-rays are also generated and may either escape from the crystal or deposit their energy via further interactions in the screen. The result of this energy cascade is the creation of a large number of electrons near the bottom of the conduction band and corresponding holes in the valence band, which can recombine directly or, more commonly, via intermediate states to give rise to the luminescence emission. In some materials such as calcium tungstate ($CaWO_4$), a commonly used phosphor in medical x-ray screens, the states

from which the emission occurs are inherent in the pure crystal. Other phosphors require added activators to produce the desired emission, for example, gadolinium oxysulfide doped with terbium ($Gd_2O_2S:Tb$), which is used in Kodak Lanex Screens (Lanex is a trademark registered by Eastman Kodak Co., Rochester, NY).

The resolution or modulation transfer function (MTF) of screen-film systems is determined primarily by the degree of scattering of photons emitted from the phosphor particles. (Although the light emission from the screen varies linearly with x-ray exposure, the film response is nonlinear. Still, in a small-amplitude approximation, the film can be treated as a linear detector, and the MTF can be used to characterize the system's spatial frequency response.) The photons emitted from the point at which an x-ray is absorbed within the screen spread as they pass through the turbid medium before escaping and exposing the film. This spread limits the system resolution. (The "blurring" of points corresponding to individual x-rays and the statistical distribution of the x-rays as mentioned above determine the appearance of the characteristic *quantum mottle* in a radiograph.) For this reason, a thicker intensifying screen usually results in a lower resolution screen-film combination; however, a thicker screen also improves x-ray absorption, which decreases system noise. For example, at the x-ray energies corresponding to the spectrum incident on the cassette in a typical 110-kVp chest examination, a pair of Lanex regular screens absorb 61 percent of the incident quanta, whereas a pair of (thinner) Lanex fine screens, used for higher resolution work, absorbs only 38 percent. This gives rise to an important trade-off in system design. Better MTF can be achieved either at the cost of system speed by using thinner screens, which then require a higher x-ray dose to expose the film, or at the cost of increased image noise by using the thinner screens with a faster (i.e., more sensitive) film. The optimum design depends on the clinical application.

Digital Technology for Projection Radiography

While screen-film technology provides high quality detection and display as well as exceptionally good archiving characteristics, there are good reasons for the tremendous amount of effort, both in industry and academia, being put into the development of electronic technologies for projection radiography. Perhaps the most obvious is compatibility with PACS. The potential benefits offered by PACS, which have been well publicized in numerous papers and conferences,[3] include reduction of lost images because data are digitally archived, easy access to patient records and examinations from multiple modalities, rapid transmission of images around a hospital, and reduction of space required for permanent archiving. Clearly, the capabilities of PACS technologies will continue to increase and the cost will continue to decrease until eventually the massive amount of information contained in projection radiographs will no longer be a limitation, at which time the fact that an acquisition system for projection radiography is digital will be a real benefit.

Currently there are no soft displays for digitized images that can provide the dynamic range and spatial resolution of film unless the user is willing to continuously manipulate contrast and level and spatially roam through an image. While soft displays will have more and more applications in the near future, dramatic improvements in the technology will be required before radiologists will have the kind of rapid access to multiple high-quality images that they now enjoy when reading from an alternator. However, this lack of soft displays will not necessarily limit the usefulness of PACS, since some laser printers currently sold for secondary imaging of computed tomography (CT), magnetic resonance imaging (MRI), digital subtraction angiography (DSA), and ultrasound data are already capable of printing images on film containing 4K × 5K 80 μm pixels with 12 bits per pixel and maximum densities approaching 3.0. While this does not match the information content of a conventional radiograph in either resolution or density range, it is probably satisfactory for many types of examinations. Furthermore, extensions of the current printer technologies would certainly occur if electronic detectors capable of providing digital data with a much higher level of image quality were to become common in the marketplace.

There are also immediate advantages offered by digital systems under development, one of which is increased exposure latitude. Most screen-film systems have a useful exposure range less than 40:1, whereas an SP system can acquire useful data over many orders of magnitude (about $10^4:1$) in exposure. This has obvious advantages such as reduction of the retake rate resulting from incorrect exposures, which could be particularly beneficial in bedside radiography, as well as provision of more information in a single exposure in examinations such as those of the chest, which can cover a large exposure range.

An additional advantage of digital systems is the decoupling of image display from image acquisition. Simple image processing, involving look-up tables that map acquired electronic levels to specific densities at the display, permit display of acquired data at any density with any contrast. Thus, for example, chests can be displayed so that either the mediastinum or the lung field covers the optimum density range for viewing. Other image processing techniques, such as edge enhancement, can also be applied to the data and may be potentially useful. As expert systems become more and more sophisticated, one expects eventually that systems that can aid in detection, and perhaps diagnosis, will also be developed. Some of these issues are discussed in more detail later in this chapter.

Storage Phosphor Technology

Imaging with SPs involves the use of screens similar in many respects to the conventional intensifying screens described above. In fact, as we will see, it is because of these similarities, both in the structure and the physical processes that occur during exposure and readout, that the potential image quality of an SP system, as measured by the detective quantum efficiency (DQE), is as good as it is relative to screen-film. Generally, SP screens consist of phosphor particles embedded in a polymer binder and coated on a flexible or rigid substrate, depending on scanner configuration. They look, for all practical purposes, like conventional screens. In general-purpose systems the SP screen is placed in a cassette and exposed by using conventional x-ray equipment. Dedicated chest and table units are also available in which the screen is an integral part of the apparatus and is not handled by the user.

The fundamental difference between the SP and the conventional screen is in the phosphors themselves. Conventional screens are designed so that as much as possible of the energy imparted to the phosphor by the x-rays is converted into "prompt" emission to form a latent image on film. SP imaging, on the other hand, makes use of a phenomenon known as *photostimulable* luminescence. This process is illustrated in Figure 6-2A. As with the conventional screens, a portion of the energy absorbed during the x-ray exposure is emitted promptly, but in addition a portion of the energy is stored in the phosphor. The latter gives rise to a *latent image* in the screen itself. Thus, no film is required in the acquisition step.

Readout of the SP latent image is accomplished by stimulating the phosphor with light (wavelength λ_1), typically in the red or near infrared for phosphors currently in use, which causes the phosphor to release the stored energy in the form of light (wavelength λ_2) of higher energy, typically in the green, blue, or near ultraviolet. Just as in the case of prompt emission from a conventional intensifying screen (or prompt emission from the SP), the intensity of the stimulated luminescence in a given area is proportional to amount of x-radiation absorbed.

In principle an image could be obtained by flooding the exposed SP screen with stimulat-

ing radiation and imaging the emitted radiation on a two-dimensional imaging detector. This is not a practical alternative, primarily because the emitted light emerges from the screen at all angles, and too much of it would be lost if imaging optics were required. High collection efficiencies are essential for good image quality. Therefore, a point by point readout scheme is generally employed, as illustrated in Figure 6-2B, which shows a simple "flatbed" flying-spot scanner. However, many other configurations can be used (e.g., helical drum scanners or flying-spot scanners with drum transports).

In the system diagrammed in Figure 6-2B, the phosphor screen sits on a translation stage, which moves it in the *page scan* or *slow scan* direction, while a laser beam, the stimulating source, is deflected across the screen in the *fast scan* direction by an oscillating mirror. Optical elements shape the beam and maintain its focus on the screen, and collection optics funnel the stimulated light emitted along the raster line up to a photodetector. Photomultiplier tubes (PMTs) are generally used as detectors because of their high sensitivities. An optical filter that selectively transmits the emission wavelength is required in front of the detector to block the laser light scattered from the screen, which can be on the order of 10^8 times as intense as the stimulated radiation itself.

As the laser beam sweeps across the screen, an analog-to-digital converter (ADC), driven by a pixel clock synchronized with the deflector, digitizes the analog signal from the detector and amplifier at the appropriate intervals to give the required number of pixels per line. Commercially available devices typically digitize at about 2000 pixels per line, although there are experimental units in use that are capable of higher resolution (about 4000 pixels per line). Once acquired in digital form, the data can be image-processed, displayed on soft displays, printed on hard copy (e.g., by using laser film printers), sent out on networks, archived, etc. Because the stimulating light actually releases the stored energy from the screen and removes the latent image, the

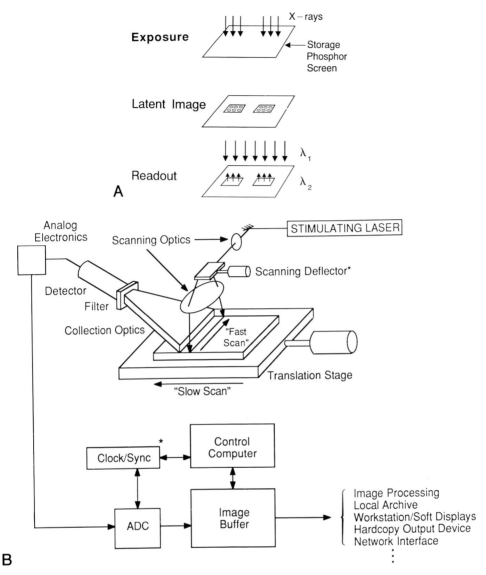

Fig. 6-2. (A) The process of photostimulable luminescence. **(B)** Diagram of an SP imaging system (see text for description).

screen is reusable. An erasing step, which involves flooding the screen with stimulating radiation, must be performed between exposures to remove any residual latent image from the previous exposure.

The physical processes that occur in the SP upon exposure to x-rays are similar to those in a conventional screen. Through a series of interactions, an absorbed x-ray produces a large number of electrons in the conduction band of the phosphor and corresponding holes in the valence band. Like a conventional phosphor, the SP must have a set of levels from which recombination can take place, giving rise to prompt emission. However, the SP also has metastable states, either inherent in the material or created by the x-rays, which can trap the electrons and thereby provide a latent image.

In many SP materials, this latent image will be stable for days (although it must still be capable of being easily stimulated for scanning and erasure). The stimulating radiation from the laser pumps the electrons into excited states, from which energy transfer can take place and recombination can occur via the same levels that produce the prompt emission. This yields the stimulated light, which is collected and digitized. The nature of the trapping and emitting states and energy transfer mechanisms depend upon the particular material. In europium-doped barium fluorobromide (BaFBr:Eu), for example, F-centers provide the electron traps and the emission is from the europium,[4-6] although there is disagreement on the precise energy transfer mechanisms involved.

A very simple argument can explain why SP image quality is basically comparable with screen-film image quality. This argument is based on two fundamental parameters controlling image quality, namely, system gain and system resolution. From a quantum noise point of view, the gain in screen-film systems can be thought of as the number of grains that develop in the film per x-ray quantum absorbed in the screen. The importance of having enough gain so that the noise in the image is primarily limited by the x-ray statistics has already been mentioned. In the SP system, the comparable gain parameter is the number of photoelectrons emitted from the photomultiplier photocathode per x-ray absorbed in the screen, electronic noise in the rest of the imaging chain being assumed to be negligible. In both systems it is often convenient to define a "noise-effective" gain that takes into account the noise created in the detection process and is thus somewhat lower than the gain defined above. (For example, in an SP system, noise associated with the amplification process in the photomultiplier dynode chain results in an effective gain that is reduced by half.)[7]

It is not surprising that the gains in the two systems are similar. For materials with comparable band gaps, the maximum number of electron/hole pairs that can be generated per absorbed x-ray is the same. Because of the prompt emission in the SP system, which is not used in the imaging process, approximately a twofold loss is incurred relative to screen-film. An additional two- or threefold loss is incurred in collecting and filtering the emission from the SP screen. However, the SP system makes up for these losses with the 20 percent quantum efficiency of the photomultiplier, compared with the film's efficiency for converting light photons into developed grains, which is on the order of 1 or 2 percent. Gain values as high as 10 for SPs have been quoted in the literature.[8,9]

As discussed earlier, the resolution in a screen-film system is largely determined by the scattering of light photons as they *exit* from the screen. In an SP system, the resolution is controlled primarily by the scattering of stimulating light photons as they *enter* the screen. Even though the diameter of the beam impinging on the SP screen can be made arbitrarily small with respect to the desired pixel size, the turbidity of the screen causes the light to scatter and spread as it penetrates, which reduces the system resolution. Again, there is a trade-off between system speed and resolution, controlled by screen thickness. If the mass densities of the phosphors are the same, comparable screen thicknesses are required for comparable x-ray absorption. The use of two thinner screens actually gives screen-film a slight resolution advantage. (Two SP screens could also be used, but this greatly increases the complexity of the acquisition system.)

The discussion of gain and resolution has obviously been simplified. The physical mechanisms occurring in both conventional phosphors and SPs vary greatly from material to material, and years of work have gone into optimizing screen efficiency. As discussed later in the chapter, practical limitations of laser power prevent reading out all the traps in the SP phosphor screen. Because the SP readout is destructive, resolution is also dependent upon laser power. Furthermore, many other noise sources affect both systems to some degree; these include variations in the number of photons produced and electrons trapped per absorbed x-ray, variations in photon escape probability as a function of depth within a screen, variations in stimulation probability as a function of depth, nonuniformities in the structure of the screens, and film grain. In addition, precise beam placement accuracy and control of laser power and transport and deflector velocities are essential to avoid noise or visual artifacts in an SP image. Nevertheless, the overall conclusion is valid: The SP system's maximum DQE, a quantitative measure of the quality of the acquired image, is comparable with (actually somewhat less than) that for the screen-film system.

Finally, it is very important to note that image quality has been compared at the *optimum* exposure for the screen-film system. Because a photomultiplier rather than a piece of film is used as the detector, the SP system has a tremendous exposure latitude compared with screen-film. Since the DQE remains high over a wide range of exposures, image information that would be lost at low exposures in the film "toe" or at high exposures in the "shoulder" is preserved in an SP system. Currently (1990), this extremely wide latitude may be SP technology's most important asset.

Historical Perspective on Storage Phosphors

The SPs used in medical radiography systems have a rich and ancient heritage in the history of scientific research. Materials that store energy and release it in the form of visible light have been known for centuries, being the object of curiosity and research from the days of alchemy.[10] Such materials were called phosphors ("light bearers"), and have been widely used to convert radiation that is invisible to the human eye into a viewable image. This process can take two basic forms: downconversion, whereby high energy radiation is absorbed and then reemitted as visible light (e.g., cathode-ray tubes), and upconversion, whereby low energy photons or thermal energy triggers the release of previously stored energy as visible light (e.g., thermoluminescence). The SP process currently used in medical radiography displays both these modes and was developed through the efforts of generations of workers.

The first preparation of phosphors came in 1603 with the Bolognian stone (barium sulfate), which would glow persistently after exposure to sunlight. By the early nineteenth century workers had observed that illumination with light of different wavelengths could influence the brightness of the energized phosphor, either enhancing or diminishing light generation. This phenomenon was used by a multitude of scientific researchers to investigate various physical processes. For instance, E. Becquerel in 1843 experimentally displayed several invisible portions of the solar spectrum by dispersing sunlight through a prism and onto an energized phosphor plate. Regions of the spectrum shorter than violet shone brightly due to downconversion of ultraviolet light, while in the spectral region beyond red the fluorescence of the phosphor was quenched by the infrared light.

Roentgen's famous discovery of x-rays in 1895 was precipitated by his observation of glowing phosphors near a cathode-ray tube. Very soon thereafter, x-rays were applied to make medical radiographs, and phosphors began to be used as downconverters to improve the sensitivity of film images. In another area, A.H. Becquerel in 1896 noted that certain uranium phosphors would glow with no optical excitation, leading to the investigation and discovery of radioactivity.

In the early twentieth century several crude attempts at phosphor imaging systems were reported.[11] During World War I Charbonneau attempted an infrared communication system, using an excited phosphor tape as the signal detector, but the performance of the materials used was too poor for any practical systems. With the advent of quantum mechanics and better understanding of fundamental processes, significant progress began to be made in fabrication of materials.

Franz Urbach in the 1920s began a systematic study of phosphor materials and the effects of additives (activators and dopants) on their characteristics.[12] He found that sensitivity could be greatly increased by using stimulation rather than quenching. During World War II research was undertaken at the University of Rochester to make SP-based infrared imaging systems for the U.S. military. It was discovered that by adding multiple dopants to certain phosphor materials (double activation) and carefully controlling their fabrication conditions, practical images were obtainable. These systems functioned by energizing the phosphor, then focusing a scene of infrared radiation on it and viewing the stimulated visible light. One such device, manufactured by Eastman Kodak Co. for the U.S. Navy, is shown in Figure 6-3. In the search for ways to energize the screens, it was noted that high-energy radiation (α particles from a small radium source) was very efficient in charging the material.

From these wartime imaging systems and increased knowledge about phosphor properties came the first suggestion of SP imaging for radiology. Berg and Kaiser proposed in 1947 that if a phosphor were energized by x-rays, the latent image might be conveniently revealed (viewed or printed on film) at a later time by stimulation with infrared light.[13] (Actually, as early as 1926, Hirsch had described a system wherein a phosphor would record x-rays and the image would later be thermally stimulated by an electric heater.[14]) This analog system thus had the basic SP concept (capture of a high-energy radiation pattern, with later revelation of the latent image by stimulation), but the state of technology development did not make it competitive with screen-film systems at the time.

In the postwar period there were significant advances in phosphor materials (driven by the television industry), electronic technology (with integrated circuits and computer systems), and lasers (which enabled rapid scanning optics). These advances made high-speed electronic imaging possible, and research at Eastman Kodak Co. led in a 1975 patent to the demonstration of the first scanned SP radiographic system[15] (Fig. 6-4). A screen composed of a thin coating of strontium sulfide powder in a binder was exposed to an x-ray pattern. By stimulating the latent image in a point-by-point serial fashion and simultaneously recording the signal generated, high quality electronic images could be generated. The screen could then be flooded with light to erase the remnant signal and reused.

SPs were proved to be linear detectors with high sensitivity and a wide latitude response as compared with conventional detector technology. The attractiveness of reusable materials and the convenience of the electronic form for storage and image manipulation were noted and became a driving force for development efforts in industry worldwide.

A review of the patent literature reveals that many companies have mounted research efforts on SPs for medical radiography: Eastman Kodak Co.; Fuji Photo Film Co., Ltd.; N.A. Philips Corp.; Konica Corp.; E.I. duPont de Nemours & Co.; 3M Co.; Agfa-Gevaert N.V.; Hitachi Ltd.; Siemens AG; Toshiba Corp.; General Electric Corp.; Kasei Optonix, Ltd.; Mitsubishi Chemical Industries, Ltd.; Nichia Corp.; GTE Products Co.; and DigiRad Corp.

The first commercial SP imaging system was announced by Fuji in 1981 under the name of the Fuji Computed Radiography System (FCR101).[8] Imaging plates were made of barium fluorobromide doped with europium (BaFBr:Eu), a very efficient material. The image was scanned out in a system consisting of a flat bed scanner with a galvanometer-deflected helium-neon laser beam, a logarithmic compressor followed by an 8-bit ADC, an image processing computer section, and a film printer to display the final image. Scan time was 90 seconds, and system cost was in the range of $500,000 to $1 million. Since the original introduction, several new models with improved performance and decreased cost have been introduced. Fuji has also licensed its system to several other companies, including Toshiba (1984), Philips Medical

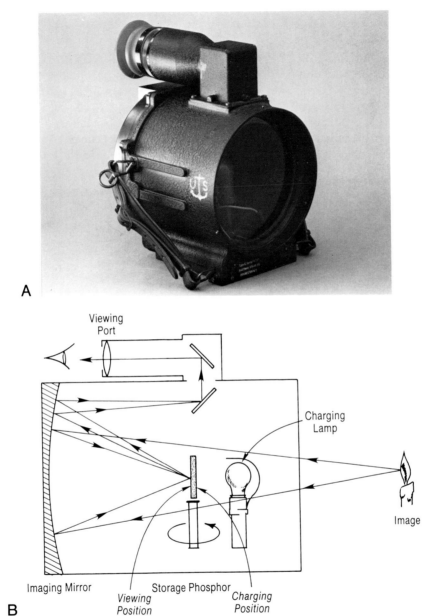

Fig. 6-3. (A & B) An infrared-sensitive night vision device using dual SP detectors. One detector is charged while the other is used for viewing.

Systems (1985), and Siemens AG (1988). At the end of 1989 nearly 300 systems had been installed worldwide, primarily in Japan.

Other announced systems include the DigiRad Filmless Radiography System (since acquired by Matrix and Agfa), which has been installed for clinical testing in two U.S. hospitals. In 1987 Konica Corp. introduced a dedicated chest unit, the Konica Direct Digitizer, which captures and scans images on an SP screen that is fixed internally in the scanning module. The system is based on a tellurium-

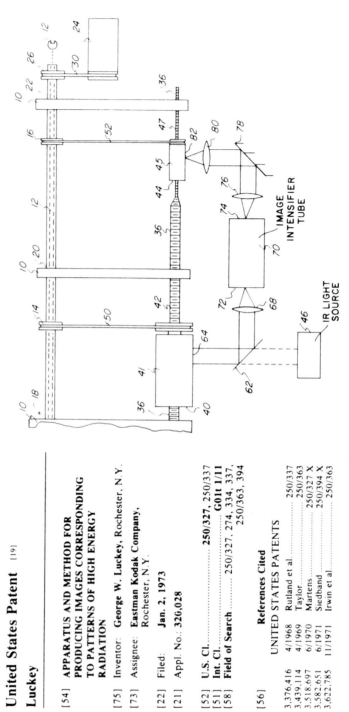

Fig. 6-4. The first scanned SP radiographic system (1975).

doped rubidium bromide material and uses an infrared laser diode to stimulate the screen. In 1986 Eastman Kodak Co. and General Electric Corp. announced a joint clinical study of an experimental high resolution SP system at the University of Pittsburgh School of Medicine to evaluate the clinical utility of SP systems. In 1988 Kodak also placed a system at Osaka University Hospital in Osaka, Japan for continuing clinical evaluations.

It also should be mentioned that SPs are being used successfully in several scientific applications other than medical projection radiography. With their linear response, high sensitivity, and wide latitude, they are attractive wherever precision detection of high energy radiation patterns is required. For instance, in x-ray diffraction studies of biologic materials, it has been found that use of SP systems permits sensitivity to be increased by more than an order of magnitude compared with conventional detectors.[16-18] Research on fundamental cellular processes, as well as on pharmaceutical drug design, is currently of great interest. When used with high intensity synchrotron sources, ultrafast exposures are possible.

Another current research area involves the analysis of genetic material by autoradiography.[19] In this application cells are processed by enzymatic agents, tagged with radioactive markers, and separated by an electrophoretic process. The resulting two-dimensional pattern of radioactive decay is used to identify the structure of the DNA sequence. Application areas include DNA "fingerprinting" for forensic testing of body materials and the human genome mapping project to catalog the human DNA sequence.

STORAGE PHOSPHOR IMAGING SYSTEMS: THEORY AND PRACTICE

This section focuses primarily on the acquisition stage of SP imaging systems and those items that influence system performance and cost. The various hardware components and materials that constitute an SP system are examined in greater detail, and their interactions are explained. The development of some powerful analytical tools for characterizing components and their interactions is also covered.

Fundamentals of System Operation

Several general characteristics of the basic SP process described in the introduction have a significant impact on the engineering design and operation of a scanner system. Some of these are the effects of destructive readout, characteristic stimulation time constants of SP materials, wide latitude acquisition, and data handling.

When the latent image is stimulated for reading, the trapped carriers are depleted and the image is erased. This means that there is only one opportunity to acquire an image, so all operating parameters (e.g., electronic gain) must be set properly. This fundamental readout process can be characterized by a stimulation curve (Fig. 6-5), which gives the amount of signal readout for a given laser exposure (exposure equals laser power multiplied by dwell time per unit area). Typical exposure energies for 50 percent readout are currently on the order of 1 mJ/cm². The stimulation curve is usually not a simple exponential function, but rather a mixture of several exponentials,[11] representing a distribution of different trapping centers in the phosphor materials.[6] As a result, the initial signal involves primarily easily stimulated sites, but at higher exposures it becomes progressively harder to stimulate the remaining higher threshold latent image.

In fact, with actual laser sources, the latent image is never completely read out — about 30 to 90 percent is typically stimulated. Therefore, additional erasure is almost always required to remove the remnant image before the screen is ready for reexposure to x-rays. It is also possible to rescan a screen and obtain further readings of the latent image, albeit with diminished signal-to-noise ratio. The operat-

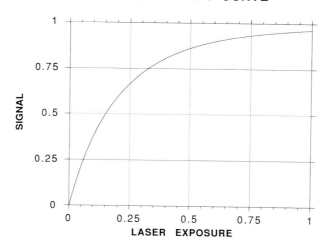

Fig. 6-5. A typical laser stimulability curve for an SP screen.

ing point (total read exposure) for a scanner may be situated on different parts of this curve, either the low power linear portion or the saturated shoulder, each with differing characteristic behavior. Normally, higher exposure and therefore higher signal level are desirable. However, signal strength and resolution are typically weakly inversely related, so unlimited increase in strength may not lead to optimum images.[20]

One subtle effect of this stimulation curve is that the generated signal is dependent on the history of laser exposure, much as is a laser print onto photographic film. As is well known for printing systems,[21] such exposure-dependent signals are susceptible to banding artifacts from intensity variations, such as transport flutter or light source fluctuations, and great care must be taken in specifying the stability of all components.

Another basic physical parameter that has an impact on system design is the fundamental response time of the stimulation process. If the stimulated luminescence has a characteristic decay time that is too long, this "afterglow" will cause a blurring that will degrade the spatial resolution of the image. Image processing can only partially compensate for this phenomenon. Time constants for stimulation vary widely with materials, but values between 0.5

to 10 μsec allow pixel sampling rates from hundreds of kilohertz to 1 MHz, corresponding to total scan times on the order of tens of seconds.

Designing a system that makes full use of the wide exposure latitude of SP screens requires careful attention to operational details. First, the screen must be properly prepared before exposure by erasing any remnant image. For instance, if a screen latitude of 10^4 is desired (latitudes in excess of 10^5 have been measured), the highest exposed portion of a previous image must be reduced to a level less than the weakest expected portion of the next exposure, since there is usually no control over image placement on a screen. To reduce latent images by more than a factor of 10^4 may require exposure to several orders of magnitude more light than that provided by the laser source during a scan. This is usually supplied by high intensity lamps in a separate erase station.

Flare, the spillover of stimulated signal from strong-signal areas into adjacent weak signal areas, is always a concern in such wide latitude systems.[18] If only 0.1 percent of the laser beam is scattered across the screen, light stimulated from high x-ray exposure areas can destroy any attempt to read the signal from nearby areas of weak latent image. Finally, the analog electronic chain must be designed to operate over this wide signal range while contributing negligible noise, and the resolution (bit depth) of the ADC must be such that its quantization intervals are smaller than the noise associated with the weakest signal while simultaneously keeping the strongest signal on scale.

Other considerations are common to all digital systems. For instance, what spatial sampling rate, or pixel size, is needed to preserve the image information content? This is an ambiguous question. Matching the resolution and information content of screen-film systems is a formidable task for any digital system, although technically possible. However, it is important to remember that the radiologist is also part of the imaging system[22] (Fig. 6-1). Thus, a more appropriate question might be: What resolution is needed to preserve the diagnostically relevant information in the image? Unfortunately, the results of diagnostic accuracy studies to determine appropriate pixel sizes for acquisition have been inconclusive, sometimes contradictory, and limited in scope.[23-25] Pixel sizes from 50 to 200 μm have been found to be adequate, depending on type of examination and pathology of interest. One practical design approach is to sample finely enough to satisfy the Nyquist criterion for the screen MTF.

As expected, these general considerations of operating an SP system lead to a set of trade-offs between the approaches and components used in a system. Referring back to Figure 6-2B, a brief description of some of these trade-offs and their characteristics follows.

SCREEN

Although the thickness of the screen is an important variable in determining SP image quality, many other factors come into play. The phosphor particle size distribution, the energy conversion efficiency, the relative amounts of phosphor and binder, and the refractive indices of the phosphor and binder also influence performance. In some cases a dye is added to the binder and/or a black backing is put between the phosphor and the substrate to absorb (i.e., prevent the spread of) the stimulating light and thereby improve MTF. Two types of commercial BaFBr:Eu screens are reported:[9] a standard screen 0.37 mm thick, and a high resolution screen 0.15 mm thick. The standard screen provides a noise-effective system gain of 3.9 (when used in the system for which it was designed) and a resolution of 1.1 lp/mm (at an MTF of 0.5), while the high-resolution screen has a gain of 2.7 and a resolution of 1.9 lp/mm (at an MTF of 0.5). The 0.37 mm BaFBr:Eu screen absorbs about 56 percent of 47-keV quanta, whereas a 0.15-mm coating absorbs about 30 percent.

LASER

Lasers are the light source of choice because of their high intensity, which is required for efficient stimulation of the SP screen within reasonable scan times. The wavelength of the laser must be matched to the simulation spectrum of the phosphor, which can range from the mid-visible to the infrared. HeNe lasers (15 to 40 mW) are commonly used, but their power levels can limit scan speeds. Higher powers are achievable with ion lasers, but these are larger and more costly. Laser diodes, which can be very efficient and compact, are used for infrared-stimulable screens. The power output from the laser must be maintained at very constant levels to prevent image artifacts. On the linear portion of the stimulation curve, specifications on allowable intensity fluctuations may be as tight as 0.1 percent, whereas on the shoulder of the curve the requirements can be considerably less. Active control, such as a feedback loop based on the light output of the laser ("noise eater"), may be required to achieve such stability.

DEFLECTOR

The deflector is the element that scans the beam across the screen. Several types can be used, depending mainly on the desired scanning rate. For relatively slow scanning (beam velocities under 5 m/s), a stationary beam may be used in conjunction with a rotating drum to scan out a helix along the curved screen surface. For scan velocities up to 50 m/s, a galvanometer-mounted mirror can be rotated to scan out a line across the screen. For even higher velocities, rotating multifaceted polygon mirrors or hologon elements are used. With the latter two, care must be taken to ensure that equal amounts of light reach the screen from each element to prevent banding artifacts. To prevent distortion such as jitter or edge waviness in an image, the beam placement error of the deflector must be kept to within fractions of a pixel dimension.

SCANNING OPTICS

Optical elements are required to focus the laser beam to a small spot on the screen and to maintain good positional control. Since the resolution of interest for medical images is usually in the range of 50 to 200 μm and because the beam size inside the screen is determined by scattering in the screen, spot size is usually not critical or diffraction-limited.

TRANSPORT

The transport is used to provide motion in the direction orthogonal to the deflector motion (slow-scan direction). It can consist of the rotary motion of a drum or the translation of a flat table. Variations in surface velocity must be kept below the detectability threshold of human observers for low-contrast objects.[21] For radiographic viewing conditions, this may mean that velocity flutter must be limited to a few tenths of 1 percent.

COLLECTION OPTICS/FILTER

Since stimulated light emitted from the screen is scattered diffusely in all directions, it must be effectively channeled to the electro-optic detector. This can be done with integrating cavities, which direct stimulated light onto the detector via diffuse or specular reflection, or with light pipes or fiberoptic bundles, which guide the light through transparent materials to the detector. High collection efficiencies are possible (80 percent efficiency has been reported for some point collectors[18]) and are essential for high signal-to-noise ratio, since this ratio is dependent upon light level. Typically, stimulation of a screen yields about 40 photons per x-ray quantum (50-keV) incident on the detector. Assuming a 2.58×10^{-7} C/kg (1 mR) exposure, a 0.1-mm pixel size scanned at a rate of 100,000 pixels per second would generate about 3×10^8 photons per second (about 10^{-10} W). (Since the laser light on the screen is on the order of tens of milliwatts, the detector must be able to detect stimulated light at levels about 10^{-8} times that of the stimulating light. This is usually achieved by use of optical filters which selectively pass only the stimulated light, attenuating the laser light by a factor of about 10^{-10}.) Uniformity of collector response across the image area is required to prevent structure artifacts in the acquired image. Finally, the scattered stimulating laser light must be controlled and prevented from reaching unintended portions of the scan. Since screens have high reflectivity (more than 80 percent typically), much of the incident light is scattered back into the scanner and can stimulate other parts of the screen, generating flare signals. These ghost images near strong exposure regions will limit the ultimate latitude of operation and must be minimized.

DETECTOR

The choice of detectors is determined by the light levels produced by the screen stimulation, which were calculated above to be fractions of a nanowatt. The only practical way at present to detect nanowatts of optical energy is to use detectors with gain (i.e., PMTs). Other devices, such as solid-state photodiodes, have too much background noise to be useful. Photomultiplier tubes have reasonable quantum efficiencies (typically 20 to 25 percent) and very good noise characteristics, with low dark currents (10^{-12} W equivalent) and relatively noise-free gain (noise figures of 2 are common). They also have large collection areas and are capable of high-speed operation. While they normally have excellent linear response to light level, at sufficiently high current levels their response can become nonlinear, which sets an upper limit for operation. The lower limit is set by their dark current, giving an operating intensity range greater than 10^3 at room temperature, which is a good match for the wide range response of the SP screen itself.

ANALOG ELECTRONICS

Once the light signal has been converted to a current by the detector, it is processed by electronic means. Amplification and filtering to limit noise are typical operations. Because such a wide range of signal strengths is possible, owing both to exposure and to anatomic variations, it is often desirable to "compress" the signal by using a logarithmic or other nonlinear converter. This puts less stress on the electronic chain but requires careful attention to avoid distortion or speed limitations. A commonly used technique to limit the required dynamic range of the electronics is to preset the electronic gain of the system to accommodate the expected signal range. This can be done by "prescanning" a screen; using a low laser power to partially read out the plate and determine the exposure level. With good design, electronics generally contributes negligible degradation to the image.

ANALOG-TO-DIGITAL CONVERTER

The ADC converts the signal voltage to digital form. It must have sufficient bit resolution to capture the smallest signal of interest and must be fast enough to sample at a rate that preserves the resolution of the image. Typically, 12-bit converters are used with linear systems, while 8- or 10-bit ADCs are used in many scanners with logarithmic converters. These systems generally use a prescan, which also helps to reduce the required number of quantization levels; without the use of prescan, more bits would be needed. Current technology allows sampling rates on ADCs to exceed 10 MHz, more than adequate for SP scan rates.

IMAGE BUFFER

A related systems issue is the size of the image data file produced by a scan. With 100-μm pixels and 12-bit resolution, more than 30 megabytes are created for a 14×17 inch image. Even with some form of data compression, handling data files of this size presents a challenge for current technology.

Performance Metrics

The basic task of the radiologist, the extraction and interpretation of the diagnostically relevant information from a complex image, is a difficult one. It uses the most complex and least understood of the human senses, vision, and yet it is done with a facility surprising to the untrained observer. Studies have reported error rates (false negative to true positive ratio) for this process in the range of 20 to 30 percent, and much work has been and is being done to identify the sources of these errors.[26,27]

The radiologic process has been divided into three main phases[28,29]: (1) search, in which the image is visually scanned to find target pathologies[30,31]; (2) detection/recognition, in which targets with sufficient signal-to-noise ratios or visual contrast are detected and organized into recognizable features or objects; and (3) decision making, in which the significance and implications for patient care of these features or objects are determined. In one study on pulmonary nodule detection roughly 30 percent of the false negative errors were attributable to the search phase, 25 percent to the detection/recognition phase, and 45 percent to the decision making phase.[29]

It is clear that our understanding of the recognition and decision making phases is still quite limited. Only recently have advances in the study of neural networks (for example, as reported by Hopfield[32]) and artificial intelligence[33] begun to hint at how the eye and brain are organized to recognize patterns and to perform diagnostic reasoning under uncertainty. Thus, if we ask how the *display* of information should be optimized to increase diagnostic accuracy, we have at present no basis in theory for predicting the answers, and we must carry out careful and sometimes lengthy experimentation to find them. Questions of this type are addressed in later sections of this chapter.

If, however, we ask how the *detection* of information should be optimized, then we can give an answer based on theory and backed by experiment. Further, the answer is very useful in specifying which quantitative measurements of image quality to make and in determining how to use these measurements to optimize hardware and materials in an SP system. Here again, it is the separation of acquisition from display afforded by digital systems that allows the functions of image capture (detection) and image display to be studied and optimized independently.

The simplest possible detection task is that of deciding whether an object of known size, shape, and position is or is not present in an image with noise. Because of its simplicity, statistical decision theory can be applied to such a task, and an "ideal" performance scale can be established.[34] Suppose we take the specific case of detecting an opaque disc, given a finite flux of transmitted photons and an imaging system with finite capabilities. Then the signal to be detected is, say, $S(x)$, a function in two dimensions describing the transmission of the disc. The signal also has a spectrum, $S(v)$, that is, it can be decomposed into spatial frequency components in a unique way. The result of applying statistical decision theory to this example is that in the "ideal" performance case the observer achieves a signal-to-noise ratio (SNR) for detecting the signal that may be determined from the equation[34]

$$\text{SNR}^2 = \int dv S^2(v) \, G^2 \, \text{MTF}^2(v)/N(v) \quad (1)$$

where $S(v)$ is the signal spectrum, G is the large-area transfer function of the imaging system, $\text{MTF}(v)$ is the modulation transfer function of the imaging system, and $N(v)$ is the noise power spectrum. We see that for detection the important performance characteristics of the imaging system are as follows:

1. *The large-area transfer function G:* In a screen-film system G is proportional to the contrast (or γ) of the film. Because of film's nonlinear response, G is not constant but rather varies strongly with exposure or density. In the case of SP radiography, G is proportional to the number of photoelectrons produced in the photodetector per absorbed x-ray. Since the output response for SP systems to x-ray exposure is linear over a wide range, G remains constant with variation in x-ray exposure.

2. *The modulation transfer function MTF(v) of the imaging system:* In screen-film systems the main physical cause of spatial blurring and MTF loss is the scattering and diffusion of the light emitted within the screen. In SP systems the analogous effect is the scattering and diffusion of the laser light that is used to read out the storage screen.

3. *The noise power spectrum N(v):* In screen-film systems this is the spectrum of density fluctuations on the film. In an SP system it is the spectrum of fluctuations in the output from the photodetector. The analysis of fluctuations in complex imaging systems is not easy,[35] and the measurement of accurate and reproducible noise spectra is a difficult art.[36] To use a simple example, if N photons are incident on an area A, then the noise, or variance, in this number is also N, assuming a Poisson process. This means that if we count the number of photons in a large number of detectors with area A, we will obtain an average result N, and the variance in the results will turn out also to be equal to N. The standard deviation in the results is $\sqrt{N}$, and the signal-to-noise ratio is $N/\sqrt{N} = \sqrt{N}$. Further, the noise in the ideal photon counting experiment is *white*, which means that the result at given spatial point is

uncorrelated with what we have found at previous points. If, instead, the photons are detected by a real imaging system, then in general we will find that the variance in the output from the imaging device is greater than the input variance, and the signal-to-noise ratio is less than at the input. Since the output signal-to-noise ratio is less than $\sqrt{N}$, the output image "appears as if" it were produced with fewer photons than were originally incident on the detector. The generalization of this concept of a noise-equivalent number of photons per unit area (NEQ) is given by the equation[37]

$$NEQ(v) = G^2 MTF^2\,(v)/N(v) \qquad (2)$$

It is noted that the NEQ above involves the same combination of parameters as does equation (1) from signal detection theory. Whereas the function $S(v)$ describes the signal spectrum for a given imaging task, $NEQ(v)$ contains the properties of the imaging system that are important for optimal performance in detection. In particular, the NEQ is the noise-equivalent number of photons per unit area that the output image appears to be "worth." The ratio of this number to the actual number Q of photons per unit area originally incident on the detector is the DQE of the detection system[37,38]:

$$DQE(v) = \frac{NEQ(v)}{Q} \qquad (3)$$

The DQE is the square of the output signal-to-noise ratio per input quantum and provides a fundamental measure of the efficiency of the imaging system. It is the DQE that we want to maximize in the detection stage of an SP system.

Let the output signal in SP detection be O, which as we have said is linearly dependent on the x-ray flux Q, with proportionality constant G:

$$O = GQ \qquad (4)$$

Then it is convenient to define and to measure the "normalized" noise power spectrum (i.e., the noise power divided by the signal squared, $N(v)/O^2$). We expect, on the basis of

theory and we find from measurements on SP materials, that the normalized noise power is well described by[9,20]

$$N(v)/O^2 = (1 + \epsilon/m + \beta)\,MTF^2/(\alpha Q) \\ + 1/(g\alpha Q) + SN \qquad (5)$$

The first term on the right side of the above equation is the (correlated) noise due to the variability in the finite number of absorbed x-ray quanta. It is directly analogous to the quantum mottle term in previous theoretical and experimental studies of screen-film systems.[39] The second term is an uncorrelated noise due to the finite number of electrons produced in the stimulated luminescence and detection processes. The last term, SN, is added to indicate that experimentally one finds a "structure noise" component in the measured noise power, which varies proportionally with the signal (as opposed to the quantum noise terms) and which becomes increasingly important at high x-ray exposures. This term is dependent on the composition and method of making the particular phosphor screen, and no adequate theoretical models for it have been published.

Taking the limit when the exposure Q is small enough that the SN term may be neglected compared with the quantum noise terms, and using equations 2 and 3, we obtain

$$DQE(v) = \cfrac{\alpha}{1 + \epsilon/m + \beta + \cfrac{1}{g\,MTF^2(v)}} \qquad (6)$$

The same expression for the DQE of SP detection has also been derived theoretically.[20] Let us discuss the physical meaning of each quantity in equation 6.

1. The numerator is the x-ray absorption α, which depends on the composition of the SP screen, the screen thickness, and the kilovoltage and filtration of the x-ray beam incident on the detector. A representative value of α for a general-purpose SP screen at 50 keV is 56 percent but x-ray absorption in SP screens has been found to decrease rapidly with kilovoltage at high kilovoltage.

2. The MTF has already been mentioned. Its main physical cause is the scattering and spreading of the stimulating (laser) light in the SP screen. The amount of light spreading is sensitive to the screen thickness, phosphor particle size distributions, and other optical parameters. By varying these parameters, an SP screen tailored to give a particular MTF response can be designed. A theoretical model for light scattering processes in SP screens has been reported,[40] and an example of calculated and measured MTF results for an SP system is given in Figure 6-6. Also, since the physical processes of light scattering are similar in both SP and conventional screens, the MTF responses of SP and screen-film detection are generally similar.

3. The quantity g is the noise-effective number of detected photoelectrons per absorbed x-ray quantum; that is, the SP system's noise-effective gain. This is the large-area response function, which for a good quantum-noise-limited detector should be much greater than unity. It should be noted that the gain directly affects the signal-to-noise performance, or DQE, at finite spatial frequencies. In fact, at high spatial frequencies, the DQE as given by equation 6 becomes directly proportional to g. Thus, an improvement in SP gain will improve the DQE at high frequencies, and this in turn will improve the ability to perform discrimination tasks involving higher resolution. As indicated earlier, a typical value for the gain in an SP is 10 or less. The analogous quantity for a screen-film system is the product of the number of photons emitted from the screen per x-ray (the quantum gain) and the DQE of the film. A value of 1,000 is typical for the quantum gain of a rare earth screen,[41] and the DQE of the film (at its optimal exposure) has a typical value of 2 to 3 percent, giving a product in the range of 20 to 30. As already mentioned, the SP gain is effectively reduced by a number of noise sources such as dark noise, photomultiplier tube amplification noise, and electronic noise. It is these noise sources that limit the exposure latitude of SP detection, whereas the exposure latitude of screen-film detection is limited by the DQE latitude of the film. Thus, since the dark noise, for example, is several orders of magnitude below the signal level at ordinary radiographic exposures, the exposure latitude of SP detection is far greater than that of screen-film detection, which is bounded by fog and film density saturation.

4. The terms $\epsilon/m + \beta$ describe the so-called excess noise, or *Swank noise*.[42,43] The term ϵ/m is the Poisson excess in the variation of the number of stored electrons created per absorbed x-ray quantum, and β describes the excess noise due to the variation in quantum gain processes within the depth of the SP screen. A theoretical analysis of these effects is given by Lubinsky et al.[20] For conventional screens the term analogous to β is due to the variation with depth of the probability of escape of the emitted light.[44] In SP screens an additional effect due to the varia-

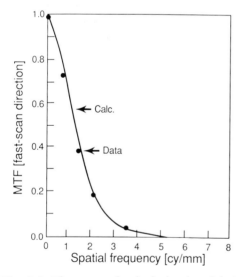

Fig. 6-6. The measured and calculated modulation transfer functions for an example (general-purpose) SP system. (From Lubinsky et al.,[40] with permission.)

tion of the stimulating laser exposure with depth contributes to β. This effect increases as the stimulating laser power decreases. As yet, very little has been published on excess noise in SPs, but preliminary results[20] indicate that SPs have a greater range of excess noise values than screen-film,[43] as illustrated in Figure 6-7. The excess noise reduces the low-frequency DQE, and thus larger excess noise means that more x-ray exposure is required for the same large-area signal-to-noise ratio.

These results are in general agreement with those reported by several other groups who have studied SP imaging from the point of view of signal-to-noise performance and DQE.[9,45,46] In addition, several contrast/detail performance studies using SPs have been conducted, along with comparisons with screen-film performance.[47-49] It is difficult to assess these studies because mixed results have been reported. Thus, one study[47] found no significant difference in threshold contrast compared with screen-film, another[48] found SP superior to screen-film in detecting small objects, and a third[49] found SP "totally inadequate" in detecting small objects, as is required, for example, in mammography.

CLINICAL APPLICATION

Throughout this chapter we have been stressing the advantages for design and analysis resulting from the separation of image acquisition and image display. In clinical practice, however, it is the total system's performance that is being tested. Moreover, this total system must include the radiologist as a key element. After all, the outcome of the medical image chain is a diagnosis, *not* an image (Fig. 6-1).

Kundel has noted that the role of observer performance in the evaluation of diagnostic imaging systems has generally been under-emphasized relative to the technical aspects of image quality.[22] While technical figures of merit are extremely important, they must somehow be related to diagnostic utility if they are to be of value in the design of new imaging systems. The relationship between technical image quality and diagnostic usefulness is often difficult to characterize, particularly for systems in which the technical level of image quality is very high. Thus, it is necessary to do extensive clinical studies to decide on the utility of new systems. For digital systems, the separation of acquisition and display

Fig. 6-7. The excess (Swank) noise in SP systems as a function of screen thickness. Also shown is the general range of excess noise values in screen-film systems. (From Lubinsky et al.,[20] with permission.)

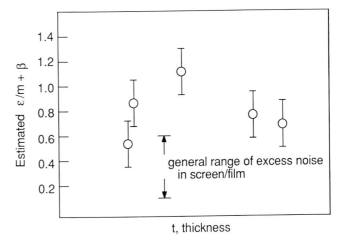

complicates such clinical studies, not only because the characteristics of the display system must be specified in addition to those of the acquisition stage, but also because of the effects of image processing.

Image Processing and the Diagnostic Process

Every digitized image, including those from SP systems, must be processed before being displayed. Often this image processing step is as simple as creating a look-up table (LUT) that maps the digital values of the image into an appropriate range for viewing on an output medium (this is essentially a window width and window level adjustment). However, more sophisticated techniques ranging from adaptive edge enhancement and smoothing to computer-aided detection and diagnosis are also being investigated. Ultimately, the value of a given image processing technique will be determined by its ability to enhance the diagnostic process, preferably by improving diagnostic accuracy, but possibly also by increasing the speed or convenience of diagnosis.

The chain connecting patient exposure to diagnosis (Fig. 6-1) contains many elements. Every link in this chain (e.g., exposure technique, scatter reduction, and detector characteristics) can affect the quality and utility of the displayed image and therefore the diagnosis. Image processing, in particular, can cause dramatic changes in the "look" of an image, changes that can challenge the radiologist's models (acquired over years of training) of what images should look like. In addition, incorrect or inappropriate image processing can create artifacts, or worse, create the appearance of disease where none exists (false positives) or cause the disappearance of disease actually present (false negatives). Thus, in evaluating the results of clinical studies of SP imaging or indeed of any other digital radiography system, the effects of image processing need to be taken into account.

Clinical Studies and Results

Evaluation of the clinical performance of projection digital radiographic systems, like that of SP imaging, can be a challenge. The high level of image quality provided by today's screen-film systems requires that large numbers of cases be collected in order to demonstrate any statistically significant improvements in diagnostic accuracy. Typically, receiver operating characteristic (ROC) methods are used as a tool in the design and analysis of such observer performance studies,[50-52] and many factors must be considered in the experimental design. Among the most important are the following:

1. *Selection of cases:* In addition to the sample size, the distribution of cases is very important. Both normal and abnormal cases must be included, and should consist of subtle cases (i.e., those that stress the system) as well as typical cases.

2. *Verification of pathology:* This is one of the most difficult aspects of performance evaluation. Observer performance must be scored on the basis of knowledge of the actual state of each patient, which can come from biopsies, autopsies, other imaging modalities, or long-term follow-up. Sometimes a panel of experts (who then are not allowed to participate in the actual study) is used to decide the "truth" in each image.

3. *Type and number of observers:* The level of training and areas of specialization of the observers can also influence the results of the study.

4. *Elimination of experimental bias:* Cases must be presented to the readers in such a way as not to influence the decision process (randomization). In addition, the effect of multiple diseases present in the same image must be dealt with in analyzing the data.

As noted above, the ability (need) to perform image processing in SP systems adds extra complexities to an already complex experiment.

In addition to such quantitative studies,

qualitative studies can be important in assessing the value of new imaging systems. Such studies, rather than being based on observer performance, are preference- or perception-based and therefore are simpler to design, require fewer images, and can be carried out more quickly. Typically, qualitative studies have been used to evaluate image quality, image processing preferences, ease of image interpretation, visibility of normal anatomy, and degree of confidence in diagnosis.[53-55]

Since the introduction of the first commercial SP systems in the early 1980s, numerous reports on their clinical use, primarily from Japan, have appeared in the literature.[53-67] The results of these studies indicate that in general the displayed image quality achievable with such systems (including the effects of image processing) is comparable with or superior to that found in current screen-film systems. However, in a few applications, most noticeably mammography, questions have been raised about the adequacy of the resolution of SP systems and the effects of screen artifacts and inappropriate image processing on final image quality.[53,57,58]

Despite the high ratings for image quality in SP systems, no quantitative evidence for statistically significant differences in diagnostic accuracy relative to conventional systems has been shown. Generally, diagnostic performance with the SP systems has been comparable with that of screen-film,[59,62-66] although it should be noted that this equivalent diagnostic accuracy was in some cases achieved at dose levels lower (by a factor of 2 to 3) than those used for the conventional exposures in these studies. This point will be addressed again below. The evaluation of diagnostic accuracy in SP systems, particularly with respect to the effects of image processing, is an area in which considerable research is still ongoing.

For the most part, the generally positive evaluations of SP image quality are attributed to two factors: the linearity and extended exposure latitude of the detector and the ability to perform image processing. The linearity and exposure latitude allow the capture and subsequent display of information that would normally fall in the toe and shoulder of the characteristic curve of most screen-film combinations. This enables more information to be obtained from a single exposure. The ability to manipulate the image data by image processing techniques brings with it the possibility of changing (for better or worse) the relative conspicuity of structures in the image. When used correctly, such processing has improved the visibility of diagnostically relevant features, leading to increased confidence in diagnosis.[53,54,58,68]

One of the positive comments made in many clinical studies of SP imaging concerns its lower dose requirements. SP imaging is *not* an inherently lower dose technique than screen-film imaging. The real advantage, which comes as a result of the extended exposure (and DQE) latitude, is the ability to use the *same* detector over a wide exposure range. It is equally possible to use screen-film systems at the lower exposure levels used in these clinical studies provided that the screen-film combination is chosen to match the exposure range. This is more difficult to do in cases involving variable or unknown exposure levels at the detector (e.g., in bedside radiography), and therefore SPs offer distinct advantages in such applications.[65]

In order to illustrate the imaging capabilities of SP imaging systems, a brief overview of four selected clinical areas, with examples of images acquired on SP systems, is given below.

CHEST IMAGING

The wide variety of diseases and the often large subject contrast make chest images one of the most difficult examinations to diagnose. The extended exposure latitude of SP systems as well as their post-processing capabilities have made them a useful tool for chest imaging.[53,54,64,65] Figure 6-8 shows a posteroanterior chest radiograph and three processed images derived from the same set of data.

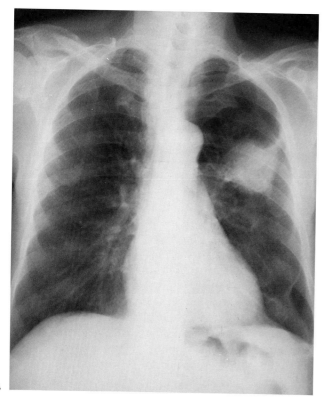

A

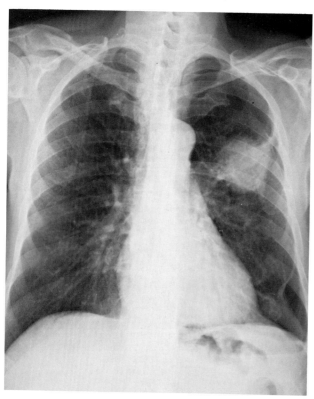

B

Fig. 6-8. A posteroanterior chest radiograph obtained with a high resolution SP imaging system (pixel size 100 μm). Four image processing variations of the same set of raw data are shown: **(A)** reference image (LUT used to give screen-film "look"); **(B)** edge-enhanced image. *(Figure continues.)*

Fig. 6-8 *(Continued).* **(C)** Edge-enhanced image with high-contrast LUT; and **(D)** edge-enhanced image with inverting LUT. (Courtesy of D. Gur, Sc.D., University of Pittsburgh, Pittsburgh, PA.)

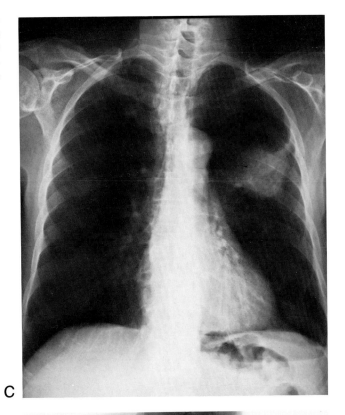

C

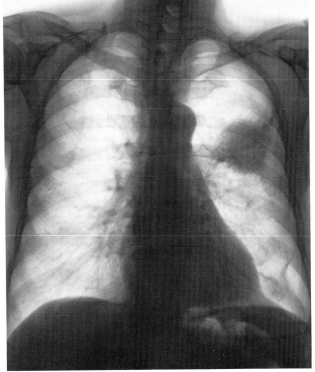

D

EXTREMITY IMAGING AND MAMMOGRAPHY

It is the area of high resolution imaging that has provided the most difficult test of SP systems' capabilities to date. There is evidence that the highest resolution available with current commercial systems (100-μm pixels) may not be sufficient to visualize fine details, such as bone trabeculae[58] or microcalcifications in breast tissue.[57] Magnification radiography has been shown to improve the resolution, although at the cost of increased tube loading and increased skin exposure.[58] It is also possible to use image processing to improve the visibility of the fine structures in images, provided, of course, that the acquisition system has sufficient DQE at these high spatial frequencies.[54,58,68] Figures 6-9 and 6-10 show examples of a foot image and a mammogram taken on an experimental, high-resolution SP imaging system (pixel size 50 μm).

RADIATION THERAPY

The use of SP imaging in the evaluation of portal images in radiation therapy is a relatively new application.[60,61,67] The extended exposure latitude of SP systems does not play a major role in this case, owing to the very low subject contrast and tighter exposure control in therapy imaging. The improvement in image quality over conventional techniques[60,61,67] is primarily due to the ability to manipulate the image data to bring out more detail from these generally poor quality images.[69] The extent of improvement has been greater for images in which air can act as a contrast medium (e.g., head, neck, chest),[55,61,67] although with analog preprocessing, improvement has also been seen in the lower contrast examinations (e.g., abdomen, pelvis).[70] Two examples of portal images taken on SPs are shown in Figures 6-11 and 6-12.

SUMMARY AND CONCLUSIONS

In this chapter we have presented a review of the technology and clinical use of SPs in medical imaging, as well as a comparison of SP systems with the screen-film systems that they are intended to replace. It can be appreciated that at present SP technology faces strong competition against established performers. The advancement of this technology is being determined as much by economic factors as by imaging performance.[71]

What are the limits on current SP systems, and what improvements can be expected? From an operational point of view, an increase in scanning speed (throughput rate) is certainly possible through the use of faster electronics and higher power lasers (both basically economic issues), but the ultimate speed limitation is the response time of the phosphor materials themselves. Current scan times can approach tens of seconds. From the standpoint of image quality, the efficiency (DQE) of current systems is fairly good, so improvements in materials and systems are not expected to provide more than a fourfold improvement in low-frequency DQE, although at higher frequencies the potential improvements may be much greater. The actual effects of such changes on diagnostic performance are still difficult to predict, and more clinical studies will be needed when and if such DQE improvements are realized.

In the overall scheme of things, however, the real technical limitation is in other parts of the digital image chain (i.e., in the PACS environment). Transmission, storage, and display of the rather large image files generated in SP systems tend to require longer periods of time than the scan operation itself. In addition, the effects on the diagnostic process of various image processing techniques need to be investigated further. Today's efforts to develop PAC systems, along with improvements in digital electronics and reductions in component costs, will eventually make the "digital

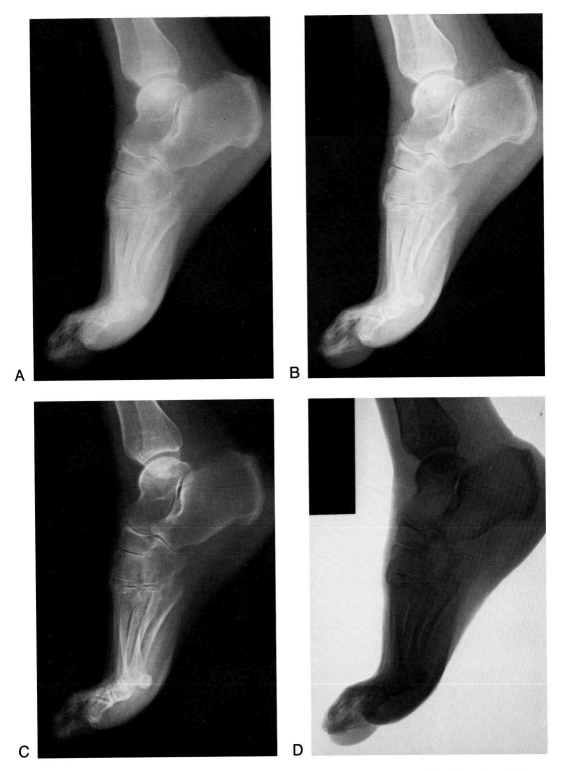

Fig. 6-9. A lateral foot image obtained with a high resolution SP imaging system (pixel size 50 μm). Four image processing variations (as in Fig. 6-8) are shown. **(A)** Reference image (LUT to give screen-film "look"); **(B)** edge-enhanced image; **(C)** edge-enhanced image with high-contrast LUT; and **(D)** edge-enhanced image with inverting LUT. (Courtesy of D. Gur, Sc.D., University of Pittsburgh, Pittsburgh, PA.)

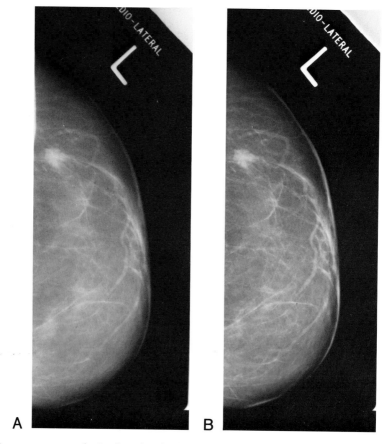

Fig. 6-10. A mammogram obtained with a high resolution SP imaging system (pixel size 50 μm). A screen-film "look-alike" image **(A)** and an edge-enhanced image **(B)** are shown. (Courtesy of D. Gur, Sc.D., , University of Pittsburgh, Pittsburgh, PA.)

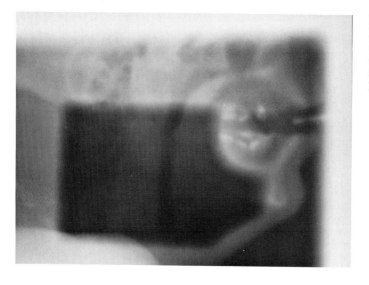

Fig. 6-11. A portal image of a lateral skull obtained with an experimental SP imaging system. (Courtesy of D. Gur, Sc.D., University of Pittsburgh, Pittsburgh, PA.)

Fig. 6-12. A portal image of a lateral pelvis obtained with an experimental SP imaging system. (The femoral head is in the radiation portal.) (Courtesy of D. Gur, Sc.D., University of Pittsburgh, Pittsburgh, PA.)

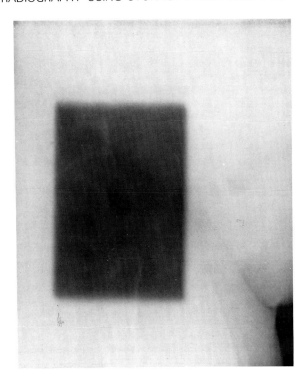

hospital" a reality. At that point, digital projection radiography will become an integral part of the radiologist's array of available imaging techniques. SP radiography is a strong candidate for inclusion in that array.

ACKNOWLEDGMENTS

We would like to thank Ken Huff for his helpful discussions on screen-film imaging and David Trauernicht and William Moore for their careful and critical reading of the manuscript. Our thanks also go to Nora Elliott for her tireless and (mostly) cheerful typing of the many revisions of this chapter and to Deborah Kenworthy for her skillful and rapid editing.

REFERENCES

1. James TH (ed): The Theory of the Photographic Process. Macmillan, New York, 1977
2. Kingsley JD: X-Ray phosphors and screens. p. 98. In Garrett DA, Bracher DA (eds): Real-Time Radiologic Imaging: Medical and Industrial Applications. ASTM Spec Tech Publ 716. Am Soc for Testing and Materials, Philadelphia, 1980
3. SPIE — International Society for Optical Engineering: Application of optical instrumentation in medicine XIV and picture archiving and communication systems (PACS IV) for medical applications. Proc SPIE 626, 1986; Medical Imaging I, Proc SPIE 767, 1987; Medical Imaging II, Proc SPIE 914, 1988
4. Takahashi K, Miyahara J, Shibahara Y: Photostimulated luminescence (PSL) and color

centers in BaFX:Eu^{2+} (X = Cl, Br, I) phosphors. J Electrochem Soc: Solid-State Sci Technol 132:1492, 1985

5. De Leeuw DM, Kovats T, Herko SP: Kinetics of photostimulated luminescence in BaFBr:Eu. J Electrochem Soc: Solid-State Sci Technol 134:491, 1987

6. Von Seggern H, Voight T, Knupfer W, Lange G: Physical model of photostimulated luminescence of x-ray irradiated BaFBr:Eu^{2+}. J Appl Phys 64:1405, 1988

7. Engstrom RW: Photomultiplier Handbook. RCA Corp., Lancaster, PA, 1980

8. Sonoda M, Takano J, Miyahara J, Kato H: Computed radiography utilizing scanning laser stimulated luminescence. Radiology 148:833, 1983

9. Hillen W, Schiebel U, Zaengel T: Imaging performance of a digital storage phosphor system. Med Phys 14:744, 1987

10. Harvey EN: A History of Luminescence. American Philosophical Society, Philadelphia, 1957

11. O'Brien B: Development of infra-red sensitive phosphors. J Opt Soc Am 36:369, 1946

12. Urbach F, Pearlman D, Hemmendinger H: On infra-red sensitive phosphors. J Opt Soc Am 36:372, 1946

13. Berg O, Kaiser H: The x-ray storage properties of the infra-red storage phosphor and application to radiography. J Appl Phys 18:343, 1947

14. Hirsch I: A new type of fluorescent screen. Radiology 7:422, 1926

15. Luckey G: U.S. Patent 3,859,527 (1975); reissued as 31,847 (1985)

16. Miyahara J, Takahashi K, Amemiya Y, et al: A new type of x-ray area detector utilizing laser stimulated luminescence. Nucl Instr Methods A246:572, 1986

17. Whiting BR, Owen JF, Rubin B: Storage phosphor x-ray diffraction detectors. Nucl Instr Methods A266:628, 1988

18. Amemiya Y, Matsushita T, Nakagawa A, et al: Design and performance of an imaging plate system for x-ray diffraction study. Nucl Instr Methods A266:645, 1988

19. Amemiya Y, Miyahara J: Imaging plate illuminates many fields. Nature 336:89, 1988

20. Lubinsky AR, Whiting BR, Owen JF: Storage phosphor system for computed radiography: Optical effects and detective quantum efficiency. Proc SPIE 767:167, 1987

21. Firth R, Kessler D, Muka E, et al: A continuous-tone laser color printer. p. 355. In SPSE Proc 3rd International Congress on Advances in Non-Impact Printing Technol: 355, 1987

22. Kundel H: Images, image quality and observer performance. Radiology 132:265, 1979

23. Lams PM, Cocklin ML: Spatial resolution requirements for digital chest radiographs: An ROC study of observer performance in selected cases. Radiology 158:11, 1986

24. MacMahon H, Vyborny CJ, Metz CE, et al: Digital radiography of subtle pulmonary abnormalities: An ROC study of the effect of pixel size on observer performance. Radiology 158:21, 1986

25. Goodman LR, Foley WD, Wilson CR, et al: Digital and conventional chest images: Observer performance with film digital radiography system. Radiology 158:27, 1986

26. Yerushalmy J: Reliability of chest radiography diagnosis of pulmonary lesions. Am J Surg 89:231, 1955

28. Garland HL: Studies on the accuracy of diagnostic procedures. AJR 82:25, 1959

28. Carmody DP, Nodine CF, Kundel HL: An analysis of perceptual and cognitive factors in radiographic interpretation. Perception 9:339, 1980

29. Kundel HL, Nodine CF, Carmody DP: Visual scanning, pattern recognition, and decision-making in pulmonary nodule detection. Invest Radiol 13:175, 1978

30. Kundel HL, LaFolette PS: Visual search patterns and experience with radiological images. Radiology 103:523, 1972

31. DeValk JPJ, Eijkman EGJ: Analysis of eye fixations during the diagnostic interpretation of chest radiographs. Med Biol Eng Comput 22:353, 1984

32. Hopfield JJ: Neural networks and physical systems with emergent collective computational abilities. Proc Natl Acad Sci USA 79:2554, 1982

33. Barr A, Feigenbaum EA: The Handbook of Artificial Intelligence. Vol. 2. William Kaufmann, Inc., Los Altos, CA, 1981, Ch. 5.

34. Wagner RF, Brown DG: Unified SNR analysis of medical imaging systems. Phys Med Biol 30:489, 1985

35. Dillon PL, Hamilton JF, Rabbani M, et al: Principles governing the transfer of signal modulation and photon noise by amplifying

and scattering mechanisms. Proc SPIE 535:130, 1985

36. Bunch PC, Van Metter R: Noise characterization and reduction in a scanning microdensitometer. Proc SPIE 767:236, 1987

37. Dainty JC, Shaw R: Image Science. Academic Press, London, 1974

38. Rose A: Vision: Human and Electronic. Plenum, New York, 1974

39. Rossman K: Modulation transfer function of radiographic systems using fluorescent screens. Phys Med Biol 9:551, 1964

40. Lubinsky AR, Owen JF, Korn DM: Storage phosphor system for computed radiography: Screen optics. Proc SPIE 626:120, 1986

41. Bunch PC, Huff KE, Shaw R, Van Metter R: Comparison of theory and experiment for the DQE of a radiographic screen-film system. Proc SPIE 535:167, 1985

42. Swank RK: Absorption and noise in x-ray phosphors. J Appl Phys 44:4199, 1967

43. Dick CE, Motz JW: Information transfer properties of x-ray fluorescent screens. Med Phys 8:337, 1981

44. Drangova M, Rowlands JA: Optical factors affecting the detective quantum efficiency of radiographic screens. Med Phys 13:150, 1986

45. Yorker JC: Photostimulated luminescence digital radiography system characterization. II: Image quality measurements. Proc SPIE 767:154, 1987

46. Klingenbeck K, Conrad B: Radiographic imaging with storage phosphors: Image quality. Siemens Forsch Entwickl Ber 16:192, 1987

47. Higashida Y, Moribe N, Hirata Y, et al: Computed radiography utilizing laser-stimulated luminescence: Detectability of simulated low-contrast radiographic objects. Comput Med Imaging Graph 12:137, 1988

48. Roehrig H, Yocky DA, Liew SC, et al: Noise and contrast performance of the Toshiba computed radiography system TCR 201. Proc SPIE 914:153, 1988

49. Shaber GS, Shlansky-Goldberg R, D'Adamo AJ: ROC detectability evaluation of a filmless digital radiographic system. Proc SPIE 914:560, 1988

50. Metz CE: Basic principles of ROC analysis. Semin Nucl Med 8:283, 1978

51. Swets JA: ROC analysis applied to the evaluation of medical imaging techniques. Invest Radiol 14:109, 1979

52. Hanley JA, McNeil BJ: The meaning and use of the area under a receiver operating characteristic (ROC) curve. Radiology 143:29, 1982

53. Milos MJ, Aberle DR, Baraff LJ, et al: Initial clinical experience with computed radiography imaging in an emergency department. Appl Radiol: 32, Jan. 1989

54. Fuhrman CR, Gur D, Good H, et al: Storage phosphor radiographs vs. conventional films: Interpreters' perceptions of diagnostic quality. AJR 150:1011, 1988

55. Fuhrman C, Deutsch M, Gur D, et al: Digital radiography using storage phosphors. p. 306. In Chiesa A, Gasparotti R, Maroldi R (eds): Proc 5th Int. Symp. on Planning of Radiological Departments: Clas International, Brescia, Italy, 1988

56. Tateno Y, Iinuma T, Takahashi M, (eds): Computed Radiography. Springer-Verlag, New York, 1987

57. Adler YT, Alcorn FS, Charters JR, et al: Computerized digital radiography in the study of breast disease. Radiology 161:328, 1986

58. Nakano Y, Hiraoka T, Togashi K, et al: Direct radiographic magnification with computed radiography. AJR 148:569, 1987

59. Fajardo LL, Hillman BJ, Hunter TB, et al: Excretory urography using computed radiography. Radiology 162:345, 1987

60. Wilenzick RM, Merritt CRB, Balter S: Megavoltage portal films using computed radiographic imaging with photostimulable phosphors. Med Phys 14:389, 1987

61. Deutsch M, Gur D, Bukovitz AG, et al: Use of storage phosphors for portal imaging in radiation therapy. Radiology 165:422, 1987

62. Megibow AJ, Beranbaum ER, Balthazar EJ, et al: Computed radiography versus film-screen radiography in double-contrast gastrointestinal radiography. Radiology 169:31, 1988

63. Shin JH, Oestmann JW, Hall DA, et al: Low-dose digital imaging: Equivalence to conventional radiography in detecting subtle gastric abnormalities in a canine model. Radiology 169:347, 1988

64. Morioka C, Brown K, Dalter S, et al: Receiver operating characteristic analysis of chest radiographs with computed radiography and conventional analog films. Radiology 169:349, 1988

65. Schaefer CM, Oestmann JW, Greene R, et al: Comparative performance of low-dose digital

and conventional radiography in bedside chests. Radiology 169:354, 1988

66. Pond GD, Seeley GW, Yoshino MT, et al: Comparison of conventional film/screen to photostimulable imaging plate radiographs for intraoperative arteriography and cholangiography. Proc SPIE 914:138, 1988

67. Gur D, Deutsch M, Fuhrman CR, et al: The use of storage phosphors for portal imaging in radiation therapy: Therapists' perception of image quality. Med Phys 16:132, 1989

68. Smathers RL, Bush E, Drace J, et al: Mammographic microcalcifications: Detection with xerography, screen-film, and digitized film display. Radiology 159:673, 1986

69. Reinstein LE, Durham M, Tefft M, et al: Portal film quality: A multiple institutional study. Med Phys 11:555, 1984

70. Weiser JC, Gur D, Deutsch M: Storage phosphor imaging in radiation therapy: Evaluation of analog contrast enhancement and digital unsharp masking in low-contrast portal images. Med Phys 17:122, 1990

71. Drew P: Computed radiography revisited: The revolution that never was. Diagn Imaging 7 June 1988

7

Image Compression and Reconstruction

Charles A. Kelsey

INTRODUCTION

Image compression consists of the processing, modification, and/or alteration of the image data to be stored so that it requires less storage space than the original data.[1-7] For example, a 1024 × 1024 × 12 bit image requires 12.6 million bits of storage space. A compression ratio of 5:1 will reduce this storage requirement to 2.5 million bits. In addition to smaller storage requirements, data compression also results in shorter image transmission time. This becomes very important when images must be transferred from one part of a hospital to another. A busy digital radiology department may generate 50 gigabytes (G bytes) of image data per day. The logistics of transferring, displaying, and sorting this amount of data are more than formidable. Data compression can make these tasks both manageable and practical.

TYPES OF IMAGE COMPRESSION

There are two types of data compression: one is completely reversible and is known as lossless, error-free, or reversible compression, while the other is not able to restore exactly the original image and is referred to as lossy or irreversible compression. Although the terms *lossless* and *error-free* have positive connotations and *lossy* and *irreversible* have negative connotations to radiologists, it is important to remember that screen-film systems have always produced irreversible compressions in the toe and shoulder region of the H and D curve. Information in the low exposure toe region is compressed and no information is recorded. The data in the shoulder region are likewise compressed, although in this region the information is recorded and can be retrieved by using a knowledge of the transfer characteristics of the screen-film system. Thus radiologists are acquainted with irreversible data compression in analog screen-film systems. The question, then, is not whether information is lost during the data processing and storage operations but whether the information loss significantly reduces the clinical usefulness of the image.

Reversible Compression

Reversible compression allows exact reconstruction of the original image. The two examples of reversible compression are *selective storage,* or *clipping,* and *run length coding.* Many digital techniques produce an image in the center of a rectangular matrix such that all the pixels outside the image have a value of zero. By searching for the edges of the clinical image, as shown in Figure 7-1, four parameters can be determined.[1] The value n_1 locates the side of the clinical image whose width is $(n_2 - n_1)$. Similarly, n_3 locates the top edge of the clinical image whose height is $(n_4 - n_3)$. A further compression can be achieved in computed tomographic (CT) images by reducing each pixel from 16 bits to 12 bits. The full 16 bits are required by the CT algorithm for cal-

culational accuracy, but storage of 12 bits will give 4096 gray levels.

Run length coding makes use of the fact that many areas of the clinical image have groups of pixels that are identical in value. Compression is achieved by storing the number of pixels with the same gray level and their gray level value together. In practice, run length coding starts by forming a histogram of the image. The least frequent gray level, say 64, is taken as the coding mark to indicate that the next two values give the number of pixels with the same gray level and their gray level. Because this coding scheme requires three values, there is no saving in compression unless more than three pixels have the same value. If not, the pixel value is stored. An example will help clarify this scheme.

EXAMPLE OF RUN LENGTH CODING

The compression search program finds 32 pixels with value zero, followed by pixels with values 3, 5, 7, and 7 and then by eight pixels with value 10. The compressed data would be stored as 64 32 0 3 5 7 7 64 8 10. In this example the compression ratio for this small line of data would be 44/10, or 4.4 : 1. If the number of pixels happens to be the same as the coding mark (64 in this example), the number is divided into two parts following a preset scheme. For example, if 64 pixels had a value of 12, they would be recorded as 64 58 12 64 6 12 with the values 58 and 6 as the preselected division of the coding mark.

HUFFMAN CODING

Huffman coding is another reversible compression scheme based on coding the frequency of occurrence of the gray levels in the image.[2] A gray scale histogram of the original image is created, and the gray level of each pixel is assigned on the basis of a series of logical steps. Huffman coding compression ratios depend on the composition of the image, but ratios of 2 : 1 can typically be achieved. It is possible to combine both run length coding

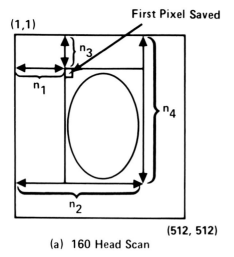

Fig. 7-1. An example of reversible compression by clipping the unused border from around the central image. (From Huang,[1] with permission.)

(1,1)

First Pixel Saved

n_3

n_1

n_4

n_2

(512, 512)

(a) 160 Head Scan

and Huffman compression schemes to obtain higher lossless compression ratios. Reversible compression techniques are limited to ratios lower than about 5 : 1 for clinical images.

Irreversible Compression

Irreversible, or *lossy* compression is usually performed by using a transfer function coding. The image is transferred into the transfer domain using a unitary two-dimensional transform such as the Fourier, cosine, Karhunen-Loeve, or Hadamard. The transform data are then approximated following an image-specific compression code, which is generated according to predetermined rules. The compression code and the approximated compressed transform data are stored as a sequential one-dimensional data file for future use in retrieving the image. To reconstruct the compressed image, the compression code is used to first decode the transform data back into a two-dimensional data array. The inverse transform is then applied to the approximated transfer function to produce the reconstructed image. The reconstructed image does not exactly duplicate the original image because of the approximations introduced during the compression steps. Irreversible compression can be considered another source of noise. Irreversible compression schemes can yield compression ratios of 20 : 1 or higher on clinical images.

DIFFERENCES BETWEEN ORIGINAL AND COMPRESSED IMAGES

Lo and Huang[5] have asked: How important is the information lost during the irreversible compression steps? They digitized a chest x-ray film with a digital camera to 512 × 512 × 8 bits and then compressed it using a full-frame bit allocation technique based on a cosine transfer function. The images produced with compression ratios of 4 : 1, 7 : 1, 12 : 1, 19 : 1 and 32 : 1 are shown in Figure 7-2 and the differences between the compressed and original images are shown in Figure 7-3. One

should notice that the variance between the compressed and the original image is distributed uniformly across the image except at the two highest compression ratios, where some anatomic features are visible. In Figure 7-3 the pixel values of the difference images were magnified by a factor of 10 before display. Investigations performed using receiver operating characteristic (ROC) studies comparing observer performance on original and compressed images have found that compression ratios up to 10 : 1 have no detectable effect on observer performance.[4-7]

IMAGE COMPRESSION TIMES

Initial compression schemes required hours of computer time and were not practical to consider for clinical use. The introduction of new hardware, chips, and algorithms programmed for the hardware have reduced processing times to the order of 1 to 4 seconds per image for both compression and decompression. Such compression and decompression times mean that processing delays are no longer a major hindrance to the acceptance of digital imaging and of picture archiving and communications systems (PACS).

MEDICOLEGAL IMPLICATIONS OF LOSSY OR IRREVERSIBLE COMPRESSION

Regardless of how much or how little information is lost, irreversible compression inevitably results in a reconstructed image that contains less information than the original. Unfortunately, this loss of information will certainly become important from a medicolegal viewpoint. No matter how many scientific studies are quoted to show that radiologists have the same accuracy and observer performance values with the compressed images as with the original images, there will be some

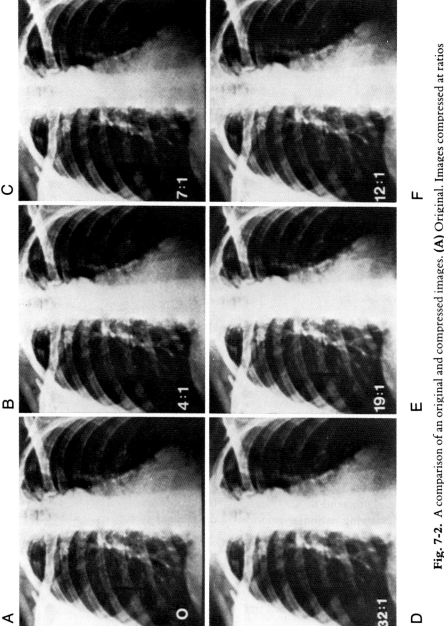

Fig. 7-2. A comparison of an original and compressed images. **(A)** Original. Images compressed at ratios of **(B)** 4:1; **(C)** 7:1; **(D)** 12:1; **(E)** 19:1; **(F)** 32:1. (From Huang,[1] with permission.)

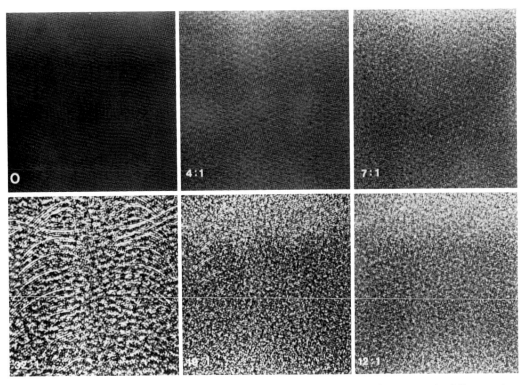

Fig. 7-3. Difference images between the original and compressed images of Fig. 7-2. The differences have been multiplied by 10. (From Huang,[1] with permission.)

who will assert that a misdiagnosis was caused by, or might have been prevented by, the lost information.

One approach to avoiding such problems is to use the original uncompressed image for the primary diagnosis and to keep it for a reasonable time (1 to 2 weeks) before storing it. In a medical center with a PACS in operation, it should be acceptable to send the compressed images to remote viewing stations if accompanied by a radiology department report based on the uncompressed images.

RADIATION DOSES

Radiation doses to most patients from a computed radiography (CR) system are the same as with modern screen-film systems. This is because modern screen-film systems are or could be quantum noise-limited. If they were not noise-limited, a higher speed system could be used. Thus there is no dose advantage in the low dose linearity characteristics of the CR system as compared with a screen-film system with the same quantum noise. In many radiology departments the techniques in general use represent a compromise and have not been optimized to lower patient radiation dose. Such systems will show a decrease in patient dose when they are switched to CR, but the same dose reduction could be achieved by choosing a faster screen-film system.

The one area in which CR does result in lower doses is pediatric radiology. Because the subjects are so small, a screen-film system requires a sufficient dose to raise the exposure levels out of the toe region of the H and D curve. The result is that in CR pediatric exposures the mAs (and dose) can be reduced fivefold as compared with a screen-film system.

REFERENCES

1. Huang HK: Elements of Digital Radiography. Prentice-Hall, Englewood Cliffs, NJ, 1987
2. Huffman DA: A method for the construction of minimum redundancy codes. Proc IRE 40:1098, 1952
3. Bramble JM, Huang HK, Murphy MD: Image data compression. Invest Radiol 23:707, 1988
4. Lo SC, Huang HK: Radiological image compression: Full frame bit allocation technique. Radiology 155:811, 1985
5. Lo SC, Huang HK: Compression of radiological images with 512, 1,024, and 2,048 matrices. Radiology 161:519, 1986
6. MacMahon H, Doi K, Sanada S, et al: Effect of data compression on diagnostic accuracy in digital chest radiography: An ROC study. Radiology 173:25, 1989
7. Halpern EJ, Levy HM, Newhouse JH, et al: Quadtree-based data compression of abdominal CT images. Invest Radiol 25:31, 1990

8

Economics of Digital Radiography

Wayne T. Stockburger

INTRODUCTION

Conversion from analog to digital radiographic imaging stimulates multiple economic concerns for providers of radiologic services. The three major concerns involve (1) capital investment, (2) personnel productivity, and (3) changes in operational expenditures. Therefore, as each aspect of digital imaging technology is evaluated for medical advantages, a simultaneous economic assessment should also occur. Regardless of whether this conversion occurs as a modular project in controlled steps or as a single dedicated effort, the transition from analog to digital radiographic image acquisition must be evaluated from an economic as well as from a clinical perspective. These assessments will prove propitious as independent observations, as well as in conjunction with each other.

Initial acquisition costs for a comprehensive digital imaging configuration are generally considered to be one-time capital expenditures. Expected useful life, as a measure of investment time, is the basis for the development of economic analysis indices. The longer the life of an investment, the greater length of time for the recovery of invested capital. Economic indices developed from useful life expectancies enable management personnel to determine fiscal effects, net annual cash flow effects, and the economic viability of the capital acquisition itself. The effective lifetime of the equipment is the primary factor in evaluating the overall cost of the system. The lifetime of complex technical equipment is usually dictated more by technical obsolescence than by the equipment actually wearing out.

In addition to economic evaluations of capital acquisition effects, conversion from analog to digital radiographic imaging must also be evaluated with respect to direct economic impacts on operational cash flows. Increased maintenance costs from the acquisition of digital imaging hardware and software are projected to be significant additions to operational expenditures. For a $2 million capital investment, increased operational costs from maintenance contracts could exceed $300,000 annually. Increased use of computerized

145

equipment as required for digital radiographic imaging necessitates increased control of environmental conditions, possibly increasing utility expenses.

The conversion from analog radiographic imaging to digital radiographic imaging via a comprehensive picture archiving and communication system (PACS) configuration does not, however, always precipitate a budgetary increase for each aspect of operations. In fact, such a conversion can produce positive as well as negative fiscal effects. The elimination of x-ray film will significantly reduce operating costs (e.g., for chemicals). Direct expenditures for film will also be reduced or eliminated.

In addition to direct economic effects associated with the conversion from analog to digital radiography, there are certain indirect economic effects which are less tangible and therefore more difficult to measure but still important. These, along with direct economic effects, should be evaluated for their individual and collective impacts on the facility. For this discussion, economic considerations associated with digital radiography will be limited to four specific categories:

Radiologist economic effects

Employee productivity effects

Operational cash flow effects

Operational profitability and economic stability effects

RADIOLOGIST ECONOMIC EFFECTS

Economic advantages that accrue to the radiologist from the application of digital technologies to radiographic image acquisition, interpretation, and management are difficult to evaluate quantitatively. Other than direct effects from improved billing efficiency, economic considerations are more often associated with indirect effects on service quality, service availability, and consumer satisfaction. A comprehensive analysis of overall economic effects on radiologist productivity must be based on a multifaceted approach concerned with both direct and indirect effects.

Radiologist economic viability is a direct function of gross billing efficiencies for services provided. While improvement of billings is not a function of digital radiography, the interface between digital imaging and radiology administrative functions through the operation of a radiology information system (RIS) will enable radiologists to maximize billing efficiencies. Net economic effects to the radiologist resulting from improved billings can be estimated from the equation

$$\text{Economic effect} = (\text{IB} + \text{RB}) \times \text{ACR} - \text{CE}$$

where   IB = increased billings
RB = recovered billings
ACR = average collection rate
CE = collection expenses

With reductions in lost charges and increases in gross billings due to improved efficiencies, positive economic indicators are produced. Total economic effect, however, is a function of workload volume, average revenue per procedure, and percentage increase to gross billings (Table 8-1). Table 8-1 emphasizes the point that a relatively small improvement in billing efficiency can result in a sig-

Table 8-1 Radiologist Economic Benefits from an 8 Percent Increase in Gross Billing Efficiency

Total Procedures	Economic Benefit[a]
10,000	$ 19,584
30,000	$ 58,752
50,000	$ 97,920
70,000	$137,088
90,000	$176,256
110,000	$215,424
130,000	$254,592
150,000	$332,928
170,000	$372,096

[a] Based on average professional billings of $40.00 per procedure, an average collection rate of 72 percent, and a 15 percent collection expense ratio.

nificant dollar increase for medium- to high-volume practices.

Indirect economic effects to radiologists through the utilization of digital imaging technologies are normally associated with the three interdependent issues of radiologist availability, service quality, and consumer satisfaction. While each of these issues is important in itself, they are functionally so fused that shortcomings in one area will severely affect the others.

For radiology groups providing services to multiple small satellite or rural facilities, traditional radiology requires extensive duplication of special modality competencies. The conversion to digital image acquisition will permit transmission of high resolution radiographic medical information from small facilities to larger, more centralized facilities, thus maximizing the availability of radiologist competencies in a group practice; specialty mixes can then be redefined to the needs of the community. The radiologist no longer needs to be physically present at multiple locations to provide services at the quality levels demanded by the local health care community.

For radiologists on call, late night emergency film readings are made more efficient through teleradiography. If a response in person is necessary, the clinicians on site need not wait for the radiologist's arrival to receive initial interpretations of preliminary films. Where additional radiographic information becomes necessary for a full diagnosis, a radiologist may authorize appropriate procedures to be performed, or at least started, before the radiologist's arrival. Waiting times for both the radiologist and the patient are reduced, and the overall medical care provided is enhanced.

Service quality with regard to the radiologist, as defined by referring clinicians and their associated patients, is normally measured in terms of accuracy of reports, availability of reports, and availability of radiographic images in direct accordance with the needs of the referring clinician. When reports are inaccurate, vague, confusing, or delayed or when the ra-diographic images are unavailable to the clinician, then service quality is judged inferior or inadequate. Use of digital imaging technologies in a comprehensive configuration will enable the radiologist to enhance service quality. Direct and immediate access to radiographic images and reports are chief among demands from clinicians. Implementation of digital image management technologies will provide simultaneous access of images to various clinician locations, while also providing access to the radiologist for consultation purposes.

Customer satisfaction concerns are applicable to economic evaluations only as they relate to reduced or enhanced utilization of radiologic services. As radiologists are able to improve the availability of their services and the accessibility of reports and images becomes a moot issue, customer satisfaction will be enhanced.

Digital imaging will not affect the problem of inaccurate, vague, and confusing reports except that the clinician will have access to the reports sooner.

EMPLOYEE PRODUCTIVITY EFFECTS

Comprehensive application of digital imaging technologies will directly affect employee productivity. In radiologic facilities that dedicate one or more technologists to the control of film quality, elimination of film will enable these employees to be assigned to other technological and quality assurance services. The conversion from analog to digital imaging as a standard process will thus produce definite positive economic effects through improved employee utilization.

Film radiography requires an estimated 5 to 7 minutes of technologist time for processing and quality control of films for each radiographic procedure. The total time consumed for these tasks, as well as the associated personnel costs, varies in direct proportion to procedure volume. Table 8-2 shows the positive

Table 8-2 Operational Costs Associated with
Technologist Time for Film Development and Quality Control

Total Procedures	Technologist Time Consumption[a] (minutes)	Full-Time Equivalents[b] (FTEs)	Personnel Costs[c]
10,000	64,800	0.59	$ 17,672
30,000	194,400	1.77	$ 53,015
50,000	324,000	2.96	$ 88,658
70,000	453,600	4.14	$124,001
90,000	583,200	5.32	$159,345
110,000	712,800	6.50	$194,688
130,000	842,400	7.68	$230,231
150,000	972,000	8.87	$265,674
170,000	1,101,600	10.05	$301,018
190,000	1,231,200	11.23	$336,361

[a] Based on 6 minutes per procedure. Time consumption totals adjusted upward by 8 percent to compensate for repeat procedures due to technologist error.
[b] One FTE equals 2,080 hours per year, adjusted upwards 13.846 percent to accommodate time lost for nonproductive factors of vacation, sick leave, jury duty, maternity leave, military leave.
[c] Personnel costs are estimated at $12.00 per technologist-hour plus 20 percent for fringe benefits of workmen's compensation, unemployment insurance, health insurance, social security taxes.

economic effects of the conversion to digital imaging that are generated by reduction in the personnel costs otherwise required for analog film processing.

The elimination of film quality control does not, however, translate into a reduction of quality assurance functions. Rather, increased information capabilities provided by digital imaging technologies expand the requirements of a comprehensive quality assurance program, which should include measures of service competencies and consumer perceptions. The quality assurance activities required by the Joint Commission on Accreditation of Healthcare Organizations (JCAHO) are not reduced by conversion to digital image acquisition. Any increases in personnel productivity can be channeled in part into required quality assurance functions.[1] The use of computed radiography (CR) during portable and tabletop radiography also produces positive personnel-related economic benefits through the elimination of exposure-related repeat procedures and consequent enhancement of technologist productivity through the reduction of time occupied by such procedures.[2] Along with savings in these personnel costs, shown in

Table 8-3, are savings in the normal imaging expenditures for film, chemistry, and equipment depreciation associated with repeat procedures.

In addition to economic benefits derived from enhanced technologist productivity, the conversion to a digital imaging configuration may also stimulate productivity enhancements in transcription and clerical job functions. While digital image acquisition will not by itself produce these effects, a comprehensive PACS will lead to improved radiology support staff productivity, especially if the PACS includes integrated transcription and optical media archival capabilities.

Transcription of reports dictated by radiologist is a labor-intensive function for radiology facilities, especially if that transcription process uses typewriters or isolated microcomputer configurations. An integrated transcription feature of a PACS eliminates isolated printing of report documents and thereby enhances productivity. This enhancement does not always result in economic benefits but often translates into improved service to users.

The transformation from analog to digital image management will also have dramatic ef-

Table 8-3 Personnel Costs Associated with Portable and Tabletop Repeat Procedures

Total Procedures	Portable and Tabletop Procedures[a]	Repeats[b]	Technologist Times (minutes)[c]	Full-Time Equivalents (FTEs)[d]	Personnel Costs[e]
10,000	4,500	360	5,400	0.05	$ 1,498
30,000	13,500	1,080	16,200	0.15	$ 4,493
50,000	22,500	1,800	27,000	0.25	$ 7,488
70,000	31,500	2,520	37,800	0.35	$10,483
90,000	40,500	3,240	48,600	0.44	$13,179
110,000	49,500	3,960	59,400	0.54	$16,175
130,000	58,500	4,680	70,200	0.64	$19,170
150,000	67,500	5,400	81,000	0.74	$22,165
170,000	76,500	6,120	91,800	0.84	$25,160
190,000	85,500	6,840	102,600	0.94	$28,155

[a] Estimates, observations, and projections indicate that 45 percent or more of all radiologic procedures are performed by portable or tabletop methods.
[b] Repeat rate of 8 percent due to exposure-related factors.
[c] 15 minutes per repeat procedure.
[d] 2,080 hours per FTE, adjusted upward 13.846 percent to compensate for vacation, sick leave, maternity leave, etc.
[e] $12.00 per technologist hour plus 20 percent fringe benefits.

fects upon productivity of the radiology file room and its associated personnel. The use of some form of optical medium for archival purposes will reduce file storage requirements by over 70 percent with current compression capabilities.[3] As compression capabilities are refined, storage capabilities of optical archival media will be further increased. Reduction in archival space requirements and enhancement of archival capabilities made possible by digital research will also result in a reduction of clerical personnel requirements. However, efficient management of radiologic archival records in digital formats will require a computer orientation not commonly possessed by present file room personnel, and therefore economic impacts are difficult to estimate. These impacts will be dependent upon the availability of personnel who are knowledgeable in computer skills applicable to file room functions. Fewer file room personnel will be required but they will require higher skills and higher pay.

Identifying economic benefits from personnel productivity enhancements is a very real concern for the radiology facility contemplating transition to digital imaging. Because of the nature of technologists' functional responsibilities, economic benefits will vary with facility work load (Fig. 8-1).

CASH FLOW EFFECTS

In addition to those economic effects attributable to enhanced personnel productivity, the digitization of imaging services can also be evaluated for overall effects on net annual cash flows. Changes in operational expenditures, enhancements to personnel productivity, and refinements to gross billing activities due to conversion to digital imaging will stimulate cash flows.

Radiology facilities making the transition from analog to digital imaging services will be able to streamline billing efficiencies through the use of integrated PACS and RIS billing features. Increases in gross billings through the elimination of human errors and time-consuming manual tasks quite often result in positive effects on functional profitability. Again, as with benefits from enhancements to personnel productivity, benefits from increased billings are a function of facility work

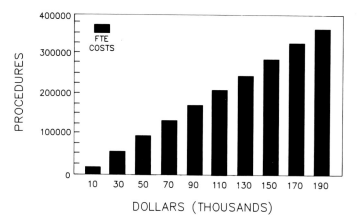

Fig. 8-1. Economic benefits from increased technologist productivity with digital radiography.

load volumes. Table 8-4 presents some representative economic benefits from a 12 percent increase in gross billing efficiency.

In addition to improved efficiency in gross billings and improvements in personnel productivity, positive net cash flow effects may also result from decreased expenditures directly associated with the installation and use of digital imaging systems. Some of the expenditure changes will be positive and some negative, and while only net effects provide insight into impact on cash flow, each specific item should be identified for overall economic evaluation (Table 8-5).

Only after the economic effects of each operational variable have been identified can an overall cash flow effect be determined. Posi-

tive economic benefits can easily be offset by negative effects, especially if depreciation and maintenance expenses are not confined to reasonable amounts. The calculation of net annual cash flow effects is vital to a comprehensive financial analysis of the transition from analog to digital radiologic imaging. This analysis of cash flow effects uses the equation

$$\text{Annual effect} = (\text{IB} + \text{RB}) \times \text{ACR} - \frac{\text{CI}}{\text{DP}}$$

$$+ \text{EBP} - \text{OCV}$$

where
- IB = increases in gross billings
- RB = recaptured gross billings
- ACR = average collection rate
- CI = capital investment
- DP = depreciation period (years)
- EBP = economic benefits for personnel productivity enhancements
- OCV = operational cost variances attributable to PACS installation

Table 8-4 Economic Benefits from a 12 Percent Increase in Gross Billing Efficiency

Total Procedures	Economic Benefit[a]
10,000	$ 66,463
30,000	$199,340
50,000	$332,316
70,000	$465,242
90,000	$598,170
110,000	$731,095
130,000	$864,022
150,000	$996,948

[a] Based on average facility billings of $90.50 per procedure and an average collection rate of 72 percent.

Table 8-5 Operational Impacts on Cash Flows From Conversion to Digital Imaging

Positive Impacts	Negative Impacts
Elimination of film expenses	Increased service costs
Elimination of chemistry expenses	Increased depreciation costs
Reduced archival floor space costs	Increased utility utilization (increased overhead)

Increased costs from PACS operations are offset by reductions of traditional expenditures. If reductions are greater than increases, then OCV will be negative indicating that savings from operations are greater than increased costs.

Example 1: Digital Imaging Cash Flows

Consider a prominent imaging facility with an annual work load volume of 90,000 procedures, which has decided to acquire a comprehensive digital PACS configuration and upon complete functional operation of this system to eliminate all analog and traditional forms of radiography from the facility. All images will be digitally acquired and directly communicated to optical archiving and reviewing workstations. Radiologists' dictations will be transcribed, and reports will be directly transferred to the hospital information system through an integration network. Initial capital expenditures are estimated to be $3.5 million, with a 7-year depreciation period. Projected changes to annual operational expenditures are as tabulated below:

Benefits from enhanced technologist productivity	$172,524
Savings from elimination of analog processing	$380,000
PACS depreciation costs	$500,000
PACS maintenance costs	$525,000
Increased revenues	$598,000
Annual cash flow effects = $598,170 − $500,000 + $172,524 + $380,000 − $525,000 = $125,000 savings	

For this imaging facility there is a significant positive annual cash flow from the conversion to digital imaging formats.

Variances in work load volumes for radiology facilities due to normal seasonal patterns, abnormal changes to referral patterns, marketplace potential, and institutional capacities provide adequate justification for the development of a comparison analysis of probable cash flows for specific work load volumes (Table 8-6).

As work load volumes fluctuate, so will net

Table 8-6 Annual Cash Flow Changes from Conversion to Comprehensive Digital Radiography

Total Procedures	Increased Revenues	Equipment Depreciation[a]	Equipment Maintenance[b]	Personnel Productivity Equivalents	Film Processing Costs[c]	Change to Cash Flow
10,000	$ 66,463	($357,143)	($375,000)	$ 19,179	$ 47,500	($617,010)
30,000	$ 199,340	($392,857)	($412,000)	$ 57,508	$138,300	($409,709)
50,000	$ 332,316	($428,572)	($450,000)	$ 96,146	$223,500	($226,610)
70,000	$ 465,242	($464,286)	($487,500)	$134,484	$303,800	($ 48,260)
90,000	$ 598,170	($500,000)	($525,000)	$172,524	$380,000	$125,694
110,000	$ 731,095	($535,000)	($562,500)	$210,863	$451,000	$295,458
130,000	$ 864,022	($571,430)	($600,000)	$249,201	$517,400	$459,193
150,000	$ 996,948	($607,143)	($637,500)	$287,839	$579,000	$619,144
170,000	$1,129,874	($642,857)	($675,000)	$326,178	$637,500	$775,695
190,000	$1,262,800	($678,572)	($712,500)	$364,516	$691,600	$927,844

[a] Initial costs of $2.5 million, with $250,000 increases in capital expenditures for every 20,000 additional procedures. Equipment costs are depreciated over a 7-year period.
[b] Equipment maintenance is calculated at 15 percent of initial capital costs.
[c] Initial film processing costs (including film, chemistry, and processor maintenance) are estimated to be $4.75 per procedure and are projected to be reduced 3 percent per 20,000 additional procedures owing to volume discounting.

annual cash flows. Conversion from traditional analog radiography to digital radiography will have a direct impact on potential billings and thereby on net annual cash flows. Evaluations of projected cash flows for multiple work load volumes indicate that smaller radiologic facilities may have more difficulty producing a net profit from operations after the conversion to a comprehensive digital imaging system (Fig. 8-2).

A mathematical equation for projection of annual cash flow effects can be developed by regression analysis.[4] Work load volumes are identified as independent variables, while projected cash flows are dependent variables. Variables from Table 8-6 have been used to construct a sample regression line for cash flow effect projections. Regression outputs indicate an X coefficient, or slope, of 8.52, an r^2 value of 0.9983, and a regression constant of −662,051 such that

$$\text{Cash flows effects} = \$8.52 \times \text{procedures} - \$662,051$$

ECONOMIC INVESTMENT VIABILITY

Positive cash flow changes generated from investment in digital imaging technologies are required for operational profitability. However, these positive cash flow effects in themselves are not adequate measures of financial viability of conversion to digital image acquisition and management. Rather, capital investments should also be evaluated according to commonly accepted methods of financial analysis for investment viability.

A net present value (NPV) analysis, performed in conjunction with cash flow evaluations, can be used to delineate overall profitability of any specific capital investment.[5] This NPV analysis will enable the facility to determine actual investment viability with respect to interest rate effects over time.

Variables required for NPV analysis are mostly obtainable from the analysis of cash flow impacts; only interest rate adjustment factors must be calculated separately. For the radiology facility evaluating the fiscal viability of transition from analog image acquisition to digital image acquisition, an NPV analysis may be performed by using the equation

$$\text{NPV} = [\sum_{n=1} ((IB + RB)_n \times (ACR)_n - OCV_n) \times PVIF_{n,i}] - CI$$

where
IB = increased billings
RB = recovered billings
ACR = average collection rate
OCV = operational cost variances
CI = capital investment
n = time period of equipment use

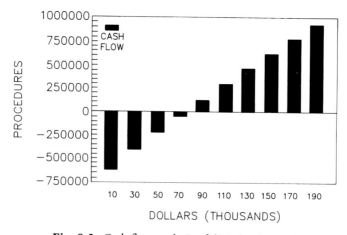

Fig. 8-2. Cash flow analysis of digital radiography.

i = capital interest rate

PVIF = Present value interest factor for n periods at i rate of interest, such that if n = 2 and i = 0.08, then $\text{PVIF}_{2,0.08} = 1/(1.08)^2 = 0.8573$

Example 2: Digital Imaging Net Present Value Analysis

A prominent imaging facility has determined that conversion to digital imaging will yield a $125,000 increase in annual cash flow. In order to determine the real value of this increase in cash flow, the imaging facility has chosen to perform a comprehensive capital investment analysis using the same statistical values as in the cash flow impact analysis. Cost of capital is estimated to be 8 percent annually, and useful life of the investment is projected to be 7 years.

For this imaging facility, economic effects over the life of the capital investment are negative. Positive annual cash flows are not substantial enough to compensate for the initial capital outlay due to the time effects of changing interest rates and monetary values.

The difference between the results of examples 1 and 2 reveals the paradox of interest rate effects on capital investments. Investment in digital imaging technologies may precipitate definite positive annual cash flows while still not providing the facility with a reasonable return on its investment, and thereby result in an investment loss.

Table 8-7 Net Present Value Analyses for Specific Work Load Volumes

Total Procedures	Net Present Value
10,000	($3,848,674)
30,000	($2,837,737)
50,000	($1,948,465)
70,000	($1,084,044)
90,000	($ 242,449)
110,000	$ 573,614
130,000	$1,365,733
150,000	$2,134,418
170,000	$2,885,407
190,000	$3,613,484

Financial variables for each net present value calculation were obtained from Tables 8-1 through 8-4. Cost of capital has been estimated to be 8 percent annually. Life of investment has been estimated to be 7 years for each work load volume.

As with the analysis of cash flow variances, NPV analyses of investment will vary with work load volume. A comparative analysis of NPVs based on procedure volumes indicates that work load volumes do exist such that positive returns on digital investments are possible (Table 8-7), and therefore a PACS becomes viable from an economic perspective. As changes in technology force prices down, this economic viability will come within the reach of smaller health care facilities.

Evaluation of projected NPVs for different work load volumes indicates that radiology facilities that perform low volumes of procedures may not receive economic benefits from conversion to digital imaging (Fig. 8-3). Until the price of digital hardware is reduced,

Year	Capital Investment	Increased Revenues	OCV	Cash Flow	PVIF	Net Effect
0	($3,500,000)	$598,170	$27,524	$625,694	1.0000	($3,500,000)
1		$598,170	$27,524	$625,694	0.9259	$ 579,330
2		$598,170	$27,524	$625,694	0.8573	$ 536,407
3		$598,170	$27,524	$625,694	0.7938	$ 496,676
4		$598,170	$27,524	$625,694	0.7350	$ 459,885
5		$598,170	$27,524	$625,694	0.6806	$ 425,847
6		$598,170	$27,524	$625,694	0.6302	$ 394,313
7		$598,170	$27,524	$625,694	0.5835	$ 364,093
					Total NPV of Investment =	($ 242,449)

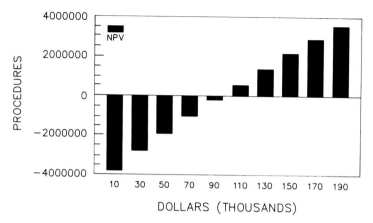

Fig. 8-3. Net present value analysis of digital radiography.

smaller radiologic facilities may be fiscally restrained from any serious consideration of digital imaging.

As with cash flow projections, a mathematical equation that will project NPVs for different work load volumes can be developed by using standard regression analysis methodologies. Work load volumes are identified as the independent variable, while projected NPVs are identified as the dependent variable. Regression analysis of the variables from Table 8-7 indicate an X coefficient, or slope of 41.152, an r^2 value of 0.9981, and a regression constant of $-4,054,060.3$, such that

$$\text{NPV} = \$41.152 \times (\text{procedures}) - \$4,054,060$$

DISCUSSION

The conversion from traditional analog to digital imaging methodologies via a comprehensive PACS configuration gives rise to several economic issues of concern. Improvements in personnel productivity through elimination of time-consuming film processing operations can have significant economic effects. Radiologists benefit from image availability at remote locations, increased con-

sumer satisfaction, and increased gross billings. Technologist productivity is enhanced through the elimination of traditional film processing, while improvements in radiology support staff translate into service improvements.

Each aspect of conversion to digital imaging has its own unique economic impacts on the various service roles of the radiology industry. Balances of negative and positive impacts can be accomplished for most medium and large volume facilities, following the development of multiple economic indicators.

The evaluation of fiscal and economic impacts of investment in digital image acquisition, archiving, display, and communication cannot be based upon any one type of analysis. Cash flow evaluations provide only indications of annual effects, while NPV analyses reveal the financial viability of the investment over time.

Overall fiscal effects are directly dependent upon work load. Large radiology facilities will experience positive cash flow effects and positive NPVs from the transition to digital imaging. Small radiology facilities may be fiscally restrained from such a transition because both cash flow effects and NPVs are likely to prove negative.

REFERENCES

1. Stockburger WT: Radiology Administration: A Business Guide. JB Lippincott, Philadelphia, 1989
2. Stockburger WT: A financial analysis of digital image acquisition for portable and table-top radiography. Radiol Management 11(1):39, 1989
3. Stockburger WT: An evaluation of the financial impacts of optical disk storage for digital radiography. Radiol Management 9(4):35, 1987
4. Summars GW, Peters WS, Armstrong CP: Basic Statistics in Business and Economics. 3rd Ed. Wadsworth Publishing Co., Belmont, CA, 1981
5. Brigham EF: Financial Management Theory and Practice. 3rd Ed. Dryden Press, Chicago, 1982

Glossary

A/D Analog to digital

ADC Analog to digital converter

Afterglow Delayed light emission after the laser readout beam has passed a point

AMBER Advanced multiple beam equalization radiography system

Black clipping Display of all signals above a cutoff level as black

CCD Charge-coupled device

Conspicuity The difference between an object and its surroundings

CR Computed radiography

CRT Cathode-ray tube

Data compression Reduction in the number of elements required to store an image

DCCR Dedicated conventional chest radiographic system

DF Digital fluorography

Digital contouring Apparent abrupt contours at interfaces caused by too few gray levels

DQE Detective quantum efficiency

DR Digital radiography

DSA Digital subtraction angiography

DTR Digital teleradiology system

FD Film digitization

II Image intensifier

Integral dose The product of the radiation dose and the mass of the tissue irradiated

Intensity histogram Histogram plot of the number of pixels having a given intensity I vs. intensity I

IP Imaging plate

Irreversible compression Data compression which cannot recover all the original data

ISDN Integrated services digital network

LAN Local area network

Latent image Image information that must be developed or processed to become visible

Logarithmic digitization Digitization of x-ray intensity using a logarithmic rather than linear scale

Lossy compression Data compression that cannot recover all the original data

Lossless compression Data compression that can recover all the original data

lp/mm line pair per millimeter

LUT Look-up table

Matrix size Size of the memory array used to store data

Mbyte One million bytes

MRI Magnetic resonance imaging

MTF Modulation transfer function

NEQ Noise equivalent quantum

NPV Net present value

Nyquist criterion A signal must be sampled at least twice the highest frequency present

PACS Picture archiving and communication system

Peak opacification Storage of the image in which the maximum opacification occurs

PMT Photomultiplier tube

PSP Photostimulable phosphor

Quantum noise Noise introduced by the quantum nature of photon production and emission

Reversible compression Data compression that can recover all the original data

RIS Radiology information system

Road mapping Storage of an image that contains the location of vessels to be catheterized during a procedure

ROC Receiver operating characteristic

SER Scanning equalization radiography

SNR Signal-to-noise ratio

SP Storage phosphor

Stochastic noise Noise generated in a random process whose average properties can be described

TCR Toshiba computed radiology system

Teleradiology The transmission and interpretation of radiologic images at a remote site

White clipping Display of all signals below a cutoff level as white

Zooming Changing the apparent magnification of an image by expanding a region of interest to fill the entire viewing screen

INDEX

Page numbers followed by f indicate figures; those followed by t indicate tables.